Nikolay Sorokin

High-Performance Reconstruction in Computer Tomography

Nikolay Sorokin

High-Performance Reconstruction in Computer Tomography

Formal Specification and Implementation

VDM Verlag Dr. Müller

Imprint

Bibliographic information by the German National Library: The German National Library lists this publication at the German National Bibliography; detailed bibliographic information is available on the Internet at http://dnb.d-nb.de.

Any brand names and product names mentioned in this book are subject to trademark, brand or patent protection and are trademarks or registered trademarks of their respective holders. The use of brand names, product names, common names, trade names, product descriptions etc. even without a particular marking in this works is in no way to be construed to mean that such names may be regarded as unrestricted in respect of trademark and brand protection legislation and could thus be used by anyone.

Cover image: www.purestockx.com

Publisher:
VDM Verlag Dr. Müller Aktiengesellschaft & Co. KG, Dudweiler Landstr. 125 a,
66123 Saarbrücken, Germany,
Phone +49 681 9100-698, Fax +49 681 9100-988,
Email: info@vdm-verlag.de

Produced in USA and UK by:
Lightning Source Inc., La Vergne, Tennessee, USA
Lightning Source UK Ltd., Milton Keynes, UK
BookSurge LLC, 5341 Dorchester Road, Suite 16, North Charleston, SC 29418, USA

ISBN: 978-3-639-02506-4

Contents

Chapter 1

Introduction

1.1 X-ray Computer Tomography

The problem of investigating the inner structure of an object was always important in different fields of science and technology. This problem is particularly actual in medicine and in non-destructive testing (NDT). Among the methods that are used for such investigations the X-ray Computer Tomography (CT) is a leading one. This is a powerful technique that deals with all types of media.

X-ray CT is based on measuring the attenuation of X-rays passed through the object. Using these measurements, called projections, acquired around the object it is possible to compute (reconstruct) the density of the original object. Mathematically projection is described by a forward Radon transform and the reconstruction is an inverse transform [1, 2, 3, 4, 5]. Depending on the measurements the reconstruction can be two- or three-dimensional. The reconstruction from projections is done using special algorithms with high operations complexity - $O(N^4)$ where N is a number of detector pixels in one detector row. Large amounts of data and high complexity of the algorithms result in long reconstruction times. For example, a 512^3-voxel volume can be reconstructed using the state-of-the-art PC in approximately five minutes [6, 7]. For the time-critical CT applications the performance is improved by parallel processing, e.g. distributing the reconstruction task between the computers connected by a network. But this solution cannot be used if the size of the system is limited, e.g. in the industrial or mobile applications. Next, the use of new, high resolution detectors introduces additional problems due to the increasing amount of data in the reconstruction process. For example [6], using detector with 1024^2 pixels the projection data occupies approximately 1.6 GB and the reconstruction of the 1024^3 volume takes 90 minutes on a single PC.

Finding alternative computing structures that can replace the multi-computer systems in special applications is an actual research topic. These structures are usually made based on special hardware, such as Digital Signal Processors (DSPs), Field Programmable Gate Arrays (FPGAs) or custom Application Specific Integrated Circuits (ASICs). Special hardware provides many possibilities to implement complex algorithms and data processing structures, and to concentrate on the optimization of critical performance parameters. Such advances as parallelization and pipelining of the operations can be easily utilized within the hardware implementation using, for example, a programmable logic basis.

1.2 Related Work

Solutions for the rapid reconstruction for the CT have been investigated for a long time. There are two main directions: software and hardware reconstruction. By software reconstruction we mean the implementation of the reconstruction using the general purpose PC systems. The reconstruction is carried out using one or several PCs connected by a network. The improvement of the reconstruction is gained by increasing the number of PCs and using optimal schemes of the parallelization. Some examples of such parallel reconstruction systems are described in works [6, 7, 8, 9, 10].

Many PCs are supplied with the graphic cards (GPUs) — very powerful stream processors: they are fully programmable, offer special pipelines for the arithmetic computations and have the special programming languages. Very important studies of the hardware reconstruction belong to the implementation of reconstruction algorithms on the base of general purpose graphic cards, e.g. work of Xu and Mueller [11] and work of Diez *et. al.* [12]. It was shown that the reconstruction on GPUs has enormous potential and possibilities.

Hardware systems, that are proposed and described in the literature, are made as special co-processor boards for PC. These hardware solutions base on different techniques, such as specialized processors, reprogrammable logic or custom logic chips.

First Very Large Scale Integration (VLSI) designs for the CT contained simple structures that have implemented only one part of the reconstruction algorithm - the backprojection step (summation) [13, 14, 15]. These were the custom designs for the two-dimensional (2D) reconstruction for the parallel-beam CT. Next studies were made by Agi *et.al.* [16, 17, 18] to combine the custom backprojectors on ASICs with DSP system. This architecture consists of the pipelined array for forward and inverse Radon transforms. The system was used for the 2D parallel- and fan-beam CT. A similar investigation, but focused on the 2D parallel-beam backprojection, was made by Trepanier *et.al.* [19]. An FPGA was used to implement the backprojection step.

Nowadays, a more practical technique is the cone-beam tomography. This type of CT has a great advantage: the time required to obtain the X-ray projections is small compared to the parallel-beam tomography. The reconstruction from cone-beam projections is a more complex task than the reconstruction from parallel-beam projections. We are aware of two works (autumn 2003) on the hardware reconstruction that deal with the three-dimensional (3D) reconstruction from cone-beam projections. Both solutions use Feldkamp cone-beam reconstruction algorithm [20]. In the first work from Terarecon [21] the 512^3 volume is reconstructed in about 128 seconds using CBR-2000 system based on XTrillion ASIC processors. The reconstruction is performed using fixed-point arithmetic. Second solution is from Mercury Computer Systems [22, 23]. An FPGA-based architecture reconstructs a volume with 512^3 voxels in approximately 39 seconds. However, no detailed information is available for these two solutions, e.g. the preciseness of the reconstruction and the information about the scalability for reconstruction of the volumes with higher number of voxels, e.g. 1024^3. This information is important for the industrial applications. Also, an ability of these systems to use new high-resolutions detectors is not mentioned.

1.3 Contribution

This book focuses on the practical implementation of the 3D CT. We provide a study of a high-speed hardware architecture for the reconstruction from cone-beam projections. A 3D reconstruction algorithm, implemented in this work, is a state-of-the-art algorithm applied in the NDT. In contrast to other works in the field of the hardware reconstruction we perform a formal description and present a specification of the parameterized hardware architecture.

A modified Feldkamp cone-beam backprojection algorithm was used for the implementation in hardware. We formalized all modifications of the algorithm. These modifications, e.g. parallelization and pipelining of the computations, significantly improve the speed of the reconstruction. Special attention was paid to the architecture of the memory system and to the schedule of the memory accesses, performed during the backprojection. All computations are performed using fixed-point arithmetic.

After the analysis of the algorithm and the specification of the parameterized hardware, we implemented the architecture in Xilinx FPGA. The impact of the different parameters on the performance, and the precision of the reconstruction were investigated. The simulations showed that a single FPGA chip with external dynamic memory is about an order of a magnitude faster than the PC system based on Intel Pentium 4,2GHz processor [6, 7]. We showed that our architecture is scalable for the reconstruction of the bigger volumes. We evaluated the hardware architecture for different number of parallel processing elements. The speed-up of the hardware architecture was obtained using theoretical and practical calculations. The influences of design parameters on the speed-up and on the scalability of the architecture were analyzed.

1.4 Structure of this book

This book is partitioned into the following chapters.

Chapter 2 presents an introduction to the field of computer tomography. It gives a basic description of the Radon transform and states the inverse problem. Methods for solving the inverse problem are described. We focus our discussion on the Filtered Backprojection, in particular on the Feldkamp cone-beam backprojection algorithm.

Chapter 3 is devoted to the practical reconstruction algorithm. We present a precise description of the reconstruction algorithm, the computation flow and make an overview of the related work.

In Chapter 4 we provide a detailed formal description of the modifications in the reconstruction algorithm. We describe now the reconstruction using the hardware approach, e.g defining the data flow between different memories and arithmetic units. We use parallelization and scheduling of the computations. Finally, we formulate the reconstruction algorithm in terms of the hardware modules.

Chapter 5 presents a detailed specification of the parameterized hardware architecture based on the formal description. We describe an implementation that performs all steps of the reconstruction from cone-beam projections: filtering of the projection data, on-line geometry computations and backprojection.

Finally, in Chapter 6 we evaluate our design and discuss the results of the implementation in Xilinx FPGA. The choice of the architecture parameters and the results of the simulations are given.

Chapter 2

Computer Tomography

In this chapter the basics of Computer Tomography reconstruction, i.e. the Radon transform and its inverse, will be discussed. We restrict this discussion to the standard problem of the reconstruction of functions from line or plane integrals. Non-standard situations, such as incomplete projections data, unknown orientations, local tomography, etc. are not dealt with.

We use the two-dimensional parallel-beam geometry to explain the Radon transform of the density function. The inverse problem will be discussed presenting different image reconstruction algorithms and comparing their features. We explain the choice of the Filtered Backprojection algorithm for our further work and describe this algorithm here. At the same time we present the discrete version of this algorithm. Introduction to Radon transform and its applications can be found in Dean's book [1]. Detailed description of the CT reconstruction from projections, different methods and techniques can be found in Herman [2], Natterer [3], Louis [4] and Kak and Slaneley [5] books and in Toft's PhD thesis [24].

2.1 Introduction and Definitions

In this part we will discuss the tomography experiment, introduce the notation and define the Radon transform.

In many applications, it is necessary to determine the distribution of some physical properties of an object (e.g. density, absorption coefficient). The value of the

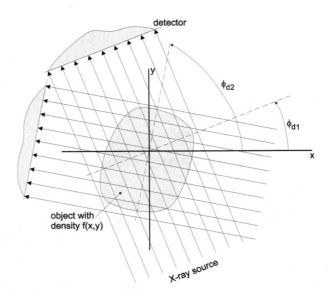

detector

ϕ_{d2}

ϕ_{d1}

y

x

object with
density f(x,y)

X-ray source

Figure 2.1: Principle of the tomography experiment: projections of an object density $f(x,y)$ are taken by measuring a set of electron beam rays for a number of different angles.

line integral of such a distribution can in certain cases be deduced from appropriate physical measurements. A set of line integrals corresponding to a particular angle of view is said to be a "projection" of the object. A finite number of such projections taken at different angles allows us to reconstruct an estimated image of the original object. Computed Tomography (CT) is a technique for imaging cross-sections of an object, placed between the X-ray source and the detector, using a series of X-ray measurements taken from different angles as shown on Figure 2.1.

Definition 1. *The density function $f : \mathbb{R} \times \mathbb{R} \to \mathbb{R}$ maps the coordinates of an object (x,y) to the density values $f(x,y)$. Outside the object $f(x,y) \equiv 0$ holds.*

We introduce the vector notation of $f(x,y)$: $f(\vec{r})$ with $\vec{r} \in \mathbb{R}^2$ and $(x,y) \equiv \vec{r}$. Through this part we will use both these notations.

Consider Figure 2.2. The intensity of the ray L from the X-ray source to the detector is attenuated by the object. If the initial intensity is I_0 and the intensity of

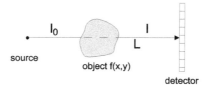

Figure 2.2: Attenuation of the ray intensity.

the ray L after the object is I, the attenuation formula is given by

$$I = I_0 \cdot e^{-\int_L f(x,y)\mathrm{d}L}.$$ (2.1.1)

We obtain the line integral value of the object function as

$$ln\frac{I_0}{I} = \int_L f(x,y)\mathrm{d}L$$ (2.1.2)

using relative attenuation I_0/I. Hence, the X-ray measurements can be considered as line-integral values using (2.1.2).

Equation (2.1.2) describes an ideal situation, when the incoming intensity is attenuated only by the object (by definition the density $f(x,y)$ outside the object is equal to zero). In practice this equation changes to an approximation due to such effects e.g. as detector sensitivity and beam-hardening. Nevertheless, for the purpose of discussing the reconstruction algorithm this is a widely accepted model [1, 2, 5].

There are different scanning geometries, which are depicted in Figure 2.3. In all of them, the object is fixed in the vertical direction. Projections are taken using two similar techniques. The first method is to fix the object and to rotate the "source-detector" system in horizontal plane. The second method is to fix the "source-detector" system and to rotate the object in horizontal plane. The first two pictures ((a),(b)) present two different two-dimensional (2D) cases. Parallel-beam projection is assumed to be a common geometry for the mathematical model presented below. Fan-beam geometry, showed on Figure 2.3(b), is another possibility of projecting, where the line integrals are measured along fans. This geometry is a more complex case, where e.g. spacing between rays must be taken into account. The 3D analogous to fan-beam is cone-beam (Figure 2.3(d)), which is widely used in CT.

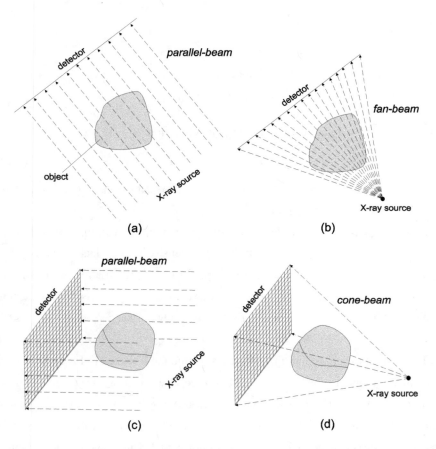

Figure 2.3: Different CT geometries: (a) parallel-beam and (b) fan-beam in 2D space, (c) parallel-beam and (d) cone-beam in 3D space.

Another type of CT geometry, widely used in medical applications, is helical scanning [25]. In this geometry the object changes it vertical position during rotation. We will not discuss this type of CT experiment here.

By ϕ_d we denote the angle between the x-axis and the normal vector from the origin to the ray L. We call this angle a projection angle. This angle changes from 0 to 2π, i.e. the object is scanned from all sides. By p we denote the distance from the origin to the ray L, i.e. every ray is defined by the pair (p, ϕ_d). A projection is formed by combining a set of line integrals for all rays for the fixed projection angle ϕ_d (see Figures 2.1 and 2.4).

Definition 2. *The function $\check{f} : \mathbb{R} \times [0, 2\pi) \to \mathbb{R}$ maps the coordinates (p, ϕ_d) to the corresponding line integral values.*

2.2 Radon Transform

The Radon transform introduces the appropriate mathematical formalism for solving a large class of practical problems, which relate to reconstructions from projections. Assume some physical probe capable of introducing projections, that approximate a cumulative measurement of some internal structure property of an object. This expresses as

$$\text{physical probe acts on } \mathbf{distribution} \Longrightarrow \textit{projection}$$

and corresponds in the case of Radon transform to

$$\text{Radon transform acts on } f(x, y) \Longrightarrow \check{f}(p, \phi_d).$$

A complete determination of $\check{f}$ requires all measurements (projections) for all angles. In applications the physical probe can be X-rays (non diffracting radiation), gamma-rays, microwaves, sound waves, etc. And these probes are used to obtain information about the wide range of internal distributions: different attenuation coefficients, densities, isotope distributions, radar brightness distributions, electron momentum in solids, etc. References to different applications of Radon transform are given in, e.g., [2, 26].

We use the 2D parallel-projection geometry as an example to define the Radon transform. For the analyses we will use Dirac delta function $\delta(x)$, which is defined as

$$\delta(x) = 0 \text{ if } x \neq 0 \text{ and } \int_{-\infty}^{\infty} \delta(x)\,dx = 1. \tag{2.2.1}$$

The 2D geometry with $\vec{r} \in \mathbb{R}^2$ is depicted on Figure 2.4. Vector $\vec{\xi}$ is a unit vector normal to the projection beam and defined as follows

$$\vec{\xi} = (\cos(\phi_d), \sin(\phi_d)).$$

Consider the ray L in the projection beam. The distance from the ray L to the origin is p (Figure 2.4(b)). The arbitrary point $(x, y) \equiv \vec{r}$ is on the ray iff

$$\vec{r} \cdot \vec{\xi} = p \tag{2.2.2}$$

holds.

By $\mathcal{R}$ we denote an operator of the Radon transform

$$\check{f} = \mathcal{R}f.$$

The Radon transform of a function $f(x, y)$ is defined as a line integral of f for all lines L defined by the parameters ϕ_d and p

$$\check{f}(p, \phi_d) = \mathcal{R}f(x, y) = \int_L f(x, y)\,dL. \tag{2.2.3}$$

Using Dirac delta function (2.2.1) and

$$p = \vec{r} \cdot \vec{\xi} = x \cdot \cos(\phi_d) + y \cdot \sin(\phi_d)$$

we rewrite Equation (2.2.3) as

$$\begin{aligned} \check{f}(p, \phi_d) &= \int_{-\infty}^{\infty} \int_{-\infty}^{\infty} f(x, y) \cdot \delta(x \cdot \cos(\phi_d) + y \cdot \sin(\phi_d) - p)\,dx\,dy \\ &= \int_{-\infty}^{\infty} f(\vec{r}) \cdot \delta(\vec{r} \cdot \vec{\xi} - p)\,d\vec{r}. \end{aligned} \tag{2.2.4}$$

In 3D the Radon transform of the density function $f(x, y, z)$ is explained using integral plane and a normal vector to it. In this case the Radon transform of the 3D

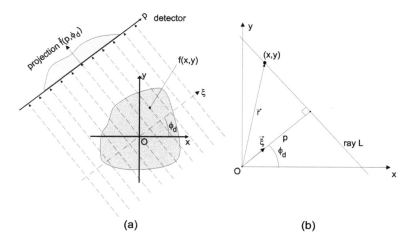

Figure 2.4: 2D experiment geometry. Coordinate system of the object is (x,y). Figure (b) depicts the coordinates in 2D space used to define Radon transform.

density function is presented by the function $\check{f}$ of 3 parameters: coordinate system of the detector (p,z) and a projection angle ϕ_d. Detailed description of the CT experiment geometries and the properties[1] of the Radon transform are described in [2, 3, 5, 24, 26, 27].

2.3 Central-Slice Theorem

One of the important properties of the Radon transform is its correspondence to the Fourier transform. This results in **central-slice theorem**[2] [3, 5, 26, 28] which will be formulated and discussed here. The reconstruction methods, that will be described in the following sections, base on this Central-slice theorem.

By (u, v) we denote Cartesian coordinates and by (q, ϕ_d) polar coordinates in the 2D Fourier space. The following equations hold

$$\begin{cases} u &= q \cdot \cos(\phi_d) \\ v &= q \cdot \sin(\phi_d). \end{cases}$$

---

[1]Linearity, Symmetry, Shifting, etc.
[2]Another name of this theorem is **"Fourier slice theorem"**

Using $\sim$ sign we denote the functions in the Fourier space. By $\mathcal{F}_n : f \mapsto \tilde{f}$ we denote the operator of n-dimensional (nD) direct Fourier transform of the nD function f, and by $\mathcal{F}_n^{-1} : \tilde{f} \mapsto f$ the operator of the nD inverse Fourier transform. Here we will use only the 1D ($\mathcal{F}_1$) and the 2D ($\mathcal{F}_2$) transforms and their inverses.

Consider functions $g(x)$ and $g(x,y)$ that are absolutely integrable[3] on $(-\infty, \infty)$ [26]. Then the 1D direct $\mathcal{F}_1 g(x)$ and inverse $\mathcal{F}_1^{-1} \tilde{g}(x)$ Fourier transforms are the functions given by

$$\tilde{g}(u) \;=\; \mathcal{F}_1 g(x) = \int_{-\infty}^{\infty} g(x)\, e^{-2\pi \imath x u}\, dx \tag{2.3.1}$$

$$g(x) \;=\; \mathcal{F}_1^{-1} \tilde{g}(u) = \int_{-\infty}^{\infty} \tilde{g}(u)\, e^{2\pi \imath x u}\, du. \tag{2.3.2}$$

For the function $g(x,y)$ we define 2D direct $\mathcal{F}_2$ and 2D inverse $\mathcal{F}_2^{-1}$ Fourier transforms as

$$\tilde{g}(u,v) \;=\; \mathcal{F}_2 g(x,y) = \int_{-\infty}^{\infty}\int_{-\infty}^{\infty} g(x,y)\, e^{-2\pi \imath (xu+yv)}\, dx\, dy \tag{2.3.3}$$

$$g(x,y) \;=\; \mathcal{F}_2^{-1} \tilde{g}(u,v) = \int_{-\infty}^{\infty}\int_{-\infty}^{\infty} \tilde{g}(u,v)\, e^{2\pi \imath (xu+yv)}\, du\, dv. \tag{2.3.4}$$

For the function defined in Cartesian coordinates (x,y), its Fourier transform will be in Cartesian coordinates (u,v) respectively. We perform 1D direct Fourier transform of a function $\check{f}(p,\phi_d)$ of the variable p and obtain the function $\check{\tilde{f}}(q,\phi_d)$ with polar coordinates (q,ϕ_d)

$$\check{\tilde{f}}(q,\phi_d) = \mathcal{F}_1 \check{f}(p,\phi_d).$$

Definition 3. *By a* **slice** *in polar coordinates* (q,ϕ_d) *we mean a ray through the origin with angle* ϕ_d.

Theorem 1. *The 1D direct Fourier transform of a projection* $\check{f}(p,\phi_d)$ *of the variable p for a fixed ϕ_d is a slice with angle ϕ_d of the 2D direct Fourier transform of the function* $f(x,y)$

$$\tilde{f}(q\cdot \cos(\phi_d), q\cdot \sin(\phi_d)) = \check{\tilde{f}}(q,\phi_d). \tag{2.3.5}$$

---

[3]i.e. $\int_{-\infty}^{\infty} |g(x)|dx < \infty$ and $\int_{-\infty}^{\infty}\int_{-\infty}^{\infty} |g(x,y)|dxdy < \infty$

The central-slice theorem holds only for the parallel-beam geometry. For the fan-beam projection geometry the projection data must be re-sorted ("rebinning" technique) into the equivalent parallel-beam projection data [5, 29, 30]. For further reading about different geometries of the Radon transform (e.g. fan-beam geometry, helical scanning) refer to [2, 5, 25].

2.4 Inverse Radon Transform

By the term *image reconstruction* or simply *reconstruction* we mean the process of forming an object image from its X-ray projections applying some algorithm.

The main aim of the Computed Tomography is the reconstruction of the object density $f(x,y)$ from the logarithmic projection data (2.1.2). It is formulated as follows:

$$\check{f} = \mathcal{R}f$$

find the density $f(x,y)$ using known values of the $\check{f}(p,\phi_d)$ $\phi_d \in [0,2\pi)$.

This is a well known mathematical inverse problem, and there exists an analytic solution, known as Radon's inversion formula [3, 4, 31]. It is not used directly in practice for several reasons. Inversion formulas (like Radon inverse formula) do not exist in all cases, e.g. when mathematical model involves weighted line integrals. However if the explicit inversion is possible, it is not evident how one can turn this analytic formula into applicable and efficient algorithm, facing a lot of problems concerning e.g. discretization and sampling.

In practice, the Radon values $\check{f}(p,\phi_d)$ are discrete and they are obtained for a finite number of projection angles. Rich mathematical apparatus is used to perform the density reconstruction from the discrete detector measurements, including Fast Fourier Transform, different types of interpolation, filtering using special functions, decompositions, etc. The goal of this part is to present an overview of some reconstruction techniques without detailed formal description. Comparing all features of these methods we will pick the optimal method of the image reconstruction, formulate a practical algorithm and describe it in continuous and discrete forms.

There are different types of reconstructed algorithms, which can be divided into two primary classes: *analytic reconstruction techniques* (transformation methods) and *iterative reconstruction techniques* (algebraic methods).

2.5 Analytic Reconstruction Techniques

These types of reconstruction methods are based on the Central-slice theorem (2.3.5) and employ different transformations, convolution, interpolations, etc., which are applied to the discrete projection values.

Analytic reconstruction methods can be subdivided into the following major classes[4]:

- Fourier based reconstruction methods, and

- Filtered Backprojection (FBP) methods.

2.5.1 Fourier Based Reconstruction Methods

Fourier based reconstruction methods (or Direct Fourier methods) are direct applications of the Central-slice theorem (2.3.5). If we apply the 1D Fourier transform to the Radon data $\check{f}(p, \phi_d)$ from the parallel-beam projections we get a 2D Fourier transform of the density function $f(x, y)$ as stated by the Central-slice theorem. *To reconstruct the density function $f(x, y)$ we apply the inverse Fourier transform* as

$$
\begin{aligned}
f(x, y) &= \mathcal{F}_2^{-1} \tilde{f}(q \cdot \cos(\phi_d), q \cdot \sin(\phi_d)) \\
&= \mathcal{F}_2^{-1} \mathcal{F}_1 \check{f}(p, \phi_d).
\end{aligned}
\tag{2.5.1}
$$

But in practice an implementation of the Equation (2.5.1) for discrete values faces a problem, namely the Central-slice theorem gives samples on a polar grid (q, ϕ_d) while the standard inverse Fourier transform requires data placed on a rectangular (Cartesian) grid (u, v). Hence, resampling to a 2D Cartesian grid is necessary. Interpolation results in such artifacts as blurring and ringing, and leads to obscuring and distorting of the reconstructed image.

---

[4]Another classification of analytic reconstruction techniques can be found in the work by Wang *et. al.* [32]; methods are divided into exact and approximate.

The artifacts can be reduced, applying such technique as gridding, which was proposed by O'Sullivan [33]. In this work the optimal gridding function was presented, and successful results were obtained when applied to the reconstruction.

Another method, called linogram method, was shown in [34]. The inversion of the Fourier data was accomplished by, first, applying the z-transform [26] and then computing the Fourier transform.

For additional information about Fourier based reconstruction methods, their modifications and applications, refer to [35, 36, 37].

The so-called "Fast image reconstruction techniques" are based on the Fourier or FBP algorithms and use different mathematical methods for the reconstruction from projections. The family of 2D domain decomposition algorithms [38, 39] and cone-beam reconstruction algorithms [40, 41] are based on a common principle. *It uses the hierarchical decomposition of the linear integral in a given direction into shorter line integral in the same direction* called "links" or "segments". Adjacent "links" are added up to create a "link" of double length. For grid size N the complete line integrals are available after $\log_2 N$ such doubling steps. Such reconstruction techniques use different interpolation methods, e.g. linear, nearest-neighbor; the accuracy of these methods and computational complexity are strongly dependent upon the specific interpolation schemes employed in the projection aggregation scheme. Extensive error analyses are done in work [42] for the multilevel domain decomposition algorithm. In this work the authors determine the correspondence of the reconstruction error to the variation of different parameters of their decomposition scheme and filtering kernels.

2.5.2 Filtered Backprojection Algorithm

Filtered Backprojection (FBP) is a frequently used algorithm for the reconstruction in CT. This algorithm is essentially a straightforward implementation of the inverse Radon transform formula. The quality of the reconstructed image is high, but this algorithm has high complexity. This is an intuitively simple algorithm: *the projection values are backprojected or "smeared back" along the line, that produced*

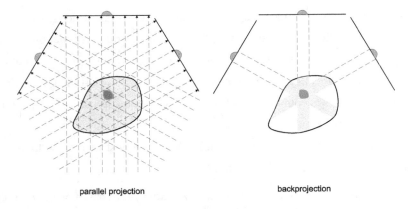

parallel projection   backprojection

Figure 2.5: Illustration to projection and backprojection in 2D case.

exactly that projection value (Figure 2.5).

Here we present the derivation of the FBP in 2D parallel-beam geometry. Let $\tilde{f}(u,v)$ be a Fourier transform of the projection data $\check{f}(p,\phi_d)$ (refer to Central-slice theorem (2.3.5)). We obtain $f(x,y)$ using the definition of the 2D inverse Fourier transform

$$f(x,y) = \mathcal{F}_2^{-1}\tilde{f}(u,v) = \int_{-\infty}^{\infty}\int_{-\infty}^{\infty}\tilde{f}(u,v)e^{2\pi i(ux+vy)}\,du\,dv.$$

This can be rewritten using $(u,v) = (q\cos(\phi_d), q\sin(\phi_d))$ and $du\,dv = q\,dq\,d\phi_d$, as

$$f(x,y) = \int_0^{2\pi}\int_{-\infty}^{\infty}\tilde{f}(q\cos(\phi_d),q\sin(\phi_d))e^{2\pi iq(x\cos(\phi_d)+y\sin(\phi_d))}q\,dq\,d\phi_d. \quad (2.5.2)$$

The Equation (2.5.2) can be split into two considering ϕ_d, first, from 0 to π, then from π to 2π,

$$\begin{aligned}
f(x,y) = \ &\int_0^{\pi}\int_0^{\infty}\tilde{f}(q\cos(\phi_d),q\sin(\phi_d))e^{2\pi iq(x\cos(\phi_d)+y\sin(\phi_d))}q\,dq\,d\phi_d \\
&+\int_0^{\pi}\int_0^{\infty}\tilde{f}(q\cos(\phi_d+\pi),q\sin(\phi_d+\pi))\cdot \\
&e^{2\pi iq(x\cos(\phi_d+\pi)+y\sin(\phi_d+\pi))}q\,dq\,d\phi_d \quad (2.5.3)
\end{aligned}$$

and we obtain

$$\begin{aligned}
f(x,y) = \ &\int_0^{\pi}\int_0^{\infty}\tilde{f}(q\cos(\phi_d),q\sin(\phi_d))e^{2\pi iq(x\cos(\phi_d)+y\sin(\phi_d))}q\,dq\,d\phi_d \\
&+\int_0^{\pi}\int_0^{\infty}\tilde{f}(-q\cos(\phi_d),-q\sin(\phi_d))\cdot
\end{aligned}$$

24

$$e^{2\pi \iota(-q)(x\cos(\phi_d)+y\sin(\phi_d))}q\,dq\,d\phi_d.$$

Next, changing the integration limits $(\infty, 0)$ to $(0, -\infty)$ in the second integral, we write

$$
\begin{aligned}
f(x,y) &= \int_0^\pi \int_0^\infty \tilde{f}(q\cos(\phi_d), q\sin(\phi_d))e^{2\pi \iota q(x\cos(\phi_d)+y\sin(\phi_d))}|q|\,dq\,d\phi_d \\
&\quad + \int_0^\pi \int_{-\infty}^0 \tilde{f}(q\cos(\phi_d), q\sin(\phi_d))e^{2\pi \iota q(x\cos(\phi_d)+y\sin(\phi_d))}|q|\,dq\,d\phi_d \\
&= \int_0^\pi \int_{-\infty}^\infty \tilde{f}(q\cos(\phi_d), q\sin(\phi_d))e^{2\pi \iota q(x\cos(\phi_d)+y\sin(\phi_d))}|q|\,dq\,d\phi_d.
\end{aligned}
$$

(2.5.4)

Let's introduce two replacements for the simplification of (2.5.4):

1. $s = x\cos(\phi_d) + y\sin(\phi_d)$, and

2. the function $W_{\phi_d} : \mathbb{R} \to \mathbb{R}$ which is expressed as

$$W_{\phi_d}(s) = \int_{-\infty}^\infty \tilde{f}(q\cos(\phi_d), q\sin(\phi_d))|q|e^{2\pi \iota q s}dq. \qquad (2.5.5)$$

Now using this simplified notation we rewrite the Equation (2.5.4)

$$f(x,y) = \int_0^\pi W_{\phi_d}(x\cos(\phi_d) + y\sin(\phi_d))\,d\phi_d. \qquad (2.5.6)$$

Equation (2.5.6) describes the backprojection for the 2D parallel-projection geometry. The term $W_{\phi_d}(s)$, given by the Equation (2.5.5), represents so called filtering operation, where the filter is given in Fourier space by $|q|$. Therefore $W_{\phi_d}(s)$ is called a "filtered projection" (projection angle ϕ_d) and the Equation (2.5.6) is called the Filtered Backprojection. In section 2.8.2 we present the technique, which avoids the interpolation of $\tilde{f}$ from polar to Cartesian grid.

One can see that the integration limits for ϕ_d are from 0 to π. This holds only for the parallel-beam geometry, because due to the even property of the delta function $\check{f}(-p, \phi_d) = \check{f}(p, \phi_d + \pi)$, i.e. this two points are situated on the same ray with angle ϕ_d. For fan-beam and cone-beam projections this does not hold [5, 27]. To reconstruct the density $f(x,y)$ the projections for all angles $\phi_d \in [0, 2\pi)$ must be obtained.

Figure 2.6 presents the reconstruction from the parallel-beam projections of the Shepp-Logan phantom [43] using Filtered Backprojection. The reconstruction was obtained using open-source software CTSim [44]. This figure visually demonstrates the reconstruction using different number of backprojection steps.

The formula for the 2D parallel-beam FBP is used only to demonstrate the back-projection technique. In applications where the real X-ray source has cone-beam radiation, some practice formulas, similar to (2.5.6) must be used. The formula for the reconstruction of the density function $f(x, y, z)$ from its cone-beam projections will be presented in section 2.8.

2.6 Iterative Reconstruction Techniques

Iterative reconstruction methods use algebraic approaches and involve matrix inversion or iterative approximations. The inverse problem is presented as a set of linear equations: every pixel of the reconstructed image has its own weighting coefficient and the sum of all elements gives the value of the line integral (projection value) for one ray of the projection. *The goal of the iterative technique is to find the solution, that represents the closest approximation to the function from which the projections were obtained.* The reconstructed image is found iteratively solving[5] the system of equations (for all rays for all projections). The values of the reconstructed density are corrected every iteration using a heuristic formula.

There are several different types of iterative reconstruction techniques, that differ in the sequence in which the corrections are made during each iteration step:

- Algebraic Reconstruction Technique (ART) [5, 45, 46, 47],

- Simultaneous Iterative Reconstruction Technique (SIRT) [45, 46],

- Simultaneous Algebraic Reconstruction Technique (SART) [5, 48].

Further descriptions of the ART methods and their practical implementation examples can be found in [5, 49, 50, 51].

---

[5]using e.g. an iterative scheme proposed by Kaczmarz (1937) to solve the system of equations

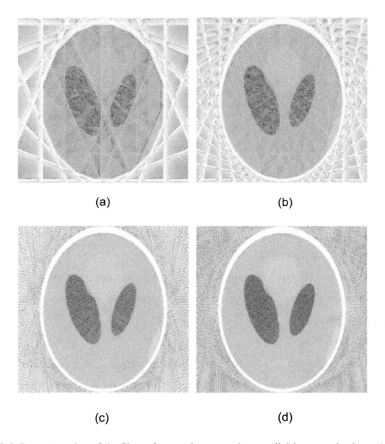

(a)   (b)

(c)   (d)

Figure 2.6: Reconstruction of the Shepp-Logan phantom using parallel-beam projections. (a) 8, (b) 16, (c) 64 and (d) 128 projections respectively. Figures from the reconstructions are obtained using the program CTSim [44].

2.7 Comparison of Different Methods

A lot of review works, e.g. [2, 5, 31, 52], include comparisons of the different methods and their variations. The conclusions in these works are dependent on the nature of the reconstructed data and particular implementation features. There is no answer what method is the best; it is likely that different methods are better for different applications.

In terms of speed and accuracy, Filtered Backprojection is preferable than other methods [32] and may produce better spatial/contrast resolution[6]. Another reason is that this reconstruction technique is more practical; it is straightforward to implement and has internal parallelism: every "filtered projection" (2.5.5) can be computed independently for every projection angle. Thus, in practice, the backprojection process can start during the measurement of the projections.

On the other hand, Fourier methods are not so straightforward and the interpolation step requires a large number of computations to avoid the introduction of artifacts into the reconstructed image.

The domain decomposition algorithms are very prospective and have good results in optimizing the backprojection. Notable speed up was reported in [38, 39], but currently these algorithms are under study to obtain error bounds and suitable mathematical models.

Compared to analytic methods the iterative reconstruction techniques are slow, because several iterations are used to obtain the suitable reconstruction result. However, iterative methods can obtain an optimal image in cases of noisy or incomplete detector data in real applications, where the analytic methods have great artifacts.

The complexity of the reconstruction algorithms can be measured in terms of the reconstruction grid size N. Normally, the grid size is equal to the number of detector pixels N in one row, so the total number of pixels in reconstructed image is N^2 for 2D case and N^3 for 3D case. The backprojection algorithm has complexity $O(N^3)$ for 2D case ($O(N^4)$ for 3D case) with the number of projections in $O(N)$.

---

[6]for the image quality discussion of the reconstruction algorithms refer to Wang's chapter "Computerized Tomography" in [52] pp.8-24.

The main advantage of the Fourier based reconstruction method is that no step of the algorithm requires more than $O(N^2 \log_2 N)$ calculations for 2D case. Domain decomposition algorithms report to have the same as Fourier-based reconstruction complexity for 2D image reconstruction, but they also require interpolation steps.

Also, the development of reconstruction algorithms is still very lively, because the new applications of CT arise almost daily and each one presents new challenges to the algorithm developers and numerical analyst scientists.

2.8 Filtered Backprojection in Detail

In the previous section we derived a set of continuous equations for the reconstruction of density function from a set of parallel projections using FBP technique. However, the infinite continuous equations for FBP can not be applied to the image reconstruction in practice for the following reasons:

- there can not be an infinite number of ϕ_d projection angles, i.e. ϕ_d will be discrete;

- the resolution of the tomography system is limited because of the finite geometrical size of the detector elements.

2.8.1 Discrete Variables and Functions

While the theoretical understanding of image reconstruction requires continuous mathematics, the practical implementation bases only on discrete variables. Most continuous variables therefore must be converted to the corresponding discrete indexed variables.

From now on we will use the following notation for the intervals of the integer variables:

$$[0:K]_\mathbb{Z} \equiv [0,K] \cap \mathbb{Z} \quad \forall K \in \mathbb{Z}.$$

Definition 4. *The number of projection angles is ϕ_{dmax} and the projections are sampled with radial interval $\Delta\phi_d$.*

Let $i_\phi \in [0 : \phi_{dmax} - 1]_{\mathbb{Z}}$ be a counter for the projections. Using Definition 4, obviously, we have

$$\phi_{di} = i_\phi \cdot \Delta\phi_d, \quad \Delta\phi_d = \frac{2\pi}{\phi_{dmax}}, \quad i_\phi \in [0 : \phi_{dmax} - 1]_{\mathbb{Z}}. \tag{2.8.1}$$

Suppose the projections contain no frequencies greater than a maximum frequency Q, i.e. the projections in Fourier space do not contain any energy outside frequency interval $(-Q, Q)$. Hence, data is sampled with interval

$$d = \frac{1}{2Q} \tag{2.8.2}$$

which is known as Nyquist condition[7] [5, 26].

In the 2D experiment geometry the detector is presented by a line of elements (similar name: "a row of detector pixels"). Assume that the number of pixels is N, where N is even. Thus, every projection will have N sample values, taken with interval d counting from center of leftmost detector element.

By $x_d \in [0 : N - 1]_{\mathbb{Z}}$ we denote a counter inside the detector row. The coordinate of sampling point p_x is

$$p_x = (x_d - N/2 + 0.5) \cdot d, \ x_d \in [0 : N - 1]_{\mathbb{Z}}, \tag{2.8.3}$$

where addition of 0.5 shifts the position of the sampling point to the center of the detector element[8]. Thus, with (p_x, ϕ_{di}) we define the discrete point with the position p_x on the projection under angle ϕ_{di}.

Definition 5. *The discrete function*

$$P_d : [0 : N - 1]_{\mathbb{Z}} \times [0 : \phi_{dmax} - 1]_{\mathbb{Z}} \to \mathbb{R}$$

maps (x_d, i_ϕ) *to the discrete values of the function* $\check{f}(p_x, \phi_{di})$

$$P_d(x_d, i_\phi) = \check{f}(p_x, \phi_{di}).$$

---

[7] or the sampling theorem in signal processing: an analog signal waveform may be uniquely reconstructed, without error, from samples taken at equal time intervals. The sampling rate must be equal to, or greater than, twice the highest frequency component in the analog signal.

[8] we assume that the elements of the detector are close together

We approximate the continuous integral equations using the following rules:

- if N_t is a number of samples of angle $\Theta \in [0, 2\pi)$, then the integral can be written using discrete variable Θ_t as

$$\int_0^{2\pi} \ldots f(\Theta) \ldots d\Theta \quad \longrightarrow \quad \frac{2\pi}{N_t} \sum_{t=0}^{N_t-1} \ldots f(\Theta_t) \ldots$$

- if N_k is a number of points in the interval $[a, b]$ and $\Delta r = (a-b)/N_k$, the integral from a to b with continuous variable r can be written using discrete variable r_k as

$$\int_b^a \ldots f(r) \ldots dr \quad \longrightarrow \quad \Delta r \sum_{k=0}^{N_k-1} \ldots f(r_k) \ldots$$

2.8.2 Filtering

Filtering is one of the important parts in the FBP. A lot of papers are devoted to filtering, discussing different filter functions, their impact on image quality and implementation of filtering. In this section we derive filtering formulas and discuss different filter types.

We rewrite the filtering projection (2.5.5) using the Central-slice theorem (2.3.5) as

$$
\begin{aligned}
W_{\phi_d}(s) &= \int_{-\infty}^{\infty} \tilde{f}(q\cos(\phi_d), q\sin(\phi_d))|q|e^{2\pi i q s} dq \\
&= \int_{-\infty}^{\infty} \left[\int_{-\infty}^{\infty} \check{f}(p, \phi_d)e^{-2\pi i q p} dp \right] |q|e^{2\pi i q s} dq \\
&= \int_{-\infty}^{\infty} \int_{-\infty}^{\infty} \check{f}(p, \phi_d)|q|e^{2\pi i q(s-p)} dp dq.
\end{aligned}
\tag{2.8.4}
$$

Let $h : \mathbb{R} \to \mathbb{R}$ be the function[9] that expresses the inverse Fourier transform of the function $|q|$

$$h(w) = \mathcal{F}_1^{-1}(|q|) = \int_{-\infty}^{\infty} |q|e^{2\pi i q w} dq. \tag{2.8.5}$$

Using function $h(w)$ with $w = s - p$ we change the Equation (2.8.4) and obtain the final formula

$$W_{\phi_d}(s) = \int_{-\infty}^{\infty} \check{f}(p, \phi_d)h(s-p)dp \tag{2.8.6}$$

---

[9]in literature this function is called sometimes a **kernel**

which is, by definition, a convolution ($*$) of two functions, $\check{f}(s,\phi_d)$ and $h(s)$.

$$W_{\phi_d}(s) = \check{f}(s,\phi_d) * h(s) \qquad (2.8.7)$$

Thus, in order to obtain the filtered projection W_{ϕ_d} the projection data must be convolved with the function $h(w)$. This convolution avoids the set of complex operations for FBP algorithm: the 1D Fourier transform of the projection data and the following interpolation from polar to Cartesian grid.

Here we present some generally accepted approximations[10] [2, 3, 5, 43, 53, 54] to the function $h(w)$ given by (2.8.5). When the projections have highest frequency Q, the function $h(w)$ can be expressed as

$$\begin{aligned} h(w) &= \int_{-Q}^{Q} |q| e^{2\pi i q w} dq \\ &= Q^2 (2 \cdot \mathrm{sinc}(2\pi w Q) - \mathrm{sinc}^2(2\pi w Q)). \end{aligned} \qquad (2.8.8)$$

where $\mathrm{sinc}(x) = \sin(x)/x$. Using $d = 1/(2Q)$ we obtain

$$h(w) = \frac{1}{2d^2} \mathrm{sinc}(\frac{\pi w}{d}) - \frac{1}{4d^2} \mathrm{sinc}(\frac{\pi w}{2d}) \qquad (2.8.9)$$

Since the projection data is measured with a sampling interval of d, the function $h(w)$ need to be known only with the same sampling interval. The samples $h(kd)$ with $k \in \mathbb{Z}$ are given by [53]

$$h(kd) = \begin{cases} 1/(4d^2) & k = 0 \\ 0 & k \text{ even} \\ -1/(k\pi d)^2 & k \text{ odd}. \end{cases} \qquad (2.8.10)$$

This filter, presented on Figure 2.7, is called the Ramachandran and Lakshminarayanan filter.

The samples of the filtering function are frequently called *"taps"* or *"filtering coefficients"*. The number of taps can be variable up to N for the case of filtering the detector row with N elements. This number of taps influences the speed and the quality of filtering in the practical applications.

---

[10]the function $|q|$ is not absolutely integrable on $(-\infty, \infty)$

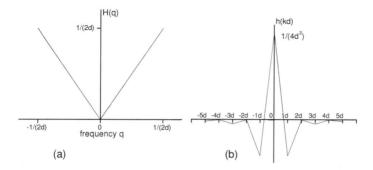

Figure 2.7: Ideal Ramp filter $|q|$ by Ramachandran and Lakshminarayanan. (a) Frequency domain, (b) discrete function $h(kd)$ from Equation (2.8.10).

The common weakness of the reconstruction algorithms is that the projection data are implicitly assumed to be noise-free (theoretically, the function is reconstructed from projections that contain no noise). However, in practice, one need to take into account the noise of the detector, the quantization errors, etc. For this purpose, there is a need to develop such special filter functions, that are less sensitive to noise. Shepp and Logan modified the Ramachandran's filter function (2.8.10) and proposed one of the low noise filter functions [43], that in discrete form is given by

$$h(kd) = \begin{cases} 4/(\pi d^2) & k = 0 \\ -4/(\pi d^2 (4k^2 - 1)) & k \in \{\pm 1, \pm 2, \pm 3, \ldots\} \end{cases} \qquad (2.8.11)$$

These discrete filter functions ((2.8.10) and (2.8.11)) are commonly used in CT applications. Other filter functions as Hamming, sinc, cosine and exponential are also used in CT for different purposes. An extensive study on filter functions for tomography have been made in the works [54, 55]. All these filters have different impact on the image reconstruction, e.g. presence of noise. The "goodness" of a filter depends on what we are looking at: some filters have bad results in places, where sharp peaks occur on projection, some filters can be noisy in general. Thus, a priori information must be used to select the suitable filter function in real CT applications.

Definition 6. *The discrete function*

$$W_d : [0 : N - 1]_{\mathbb{Z}} \times [0 : \phi_{d\,max} - 1]_{\mathbb{Z}} \to \mathbb{R}$$

maps (x_d, i_ϕ) *to the discrete filtered projections*

$$W_d(x_d, i_\phi) = W_{\phi_{d_i}}(p_x). \tag{2.8.12}$$

Using definitions of the discrete functions and variables we write the convolution (2.8.7) in discrete form (with N taps filtering function $h()$)

$$W_d(x_d, i_\phi) = W_{\phi_{d_i}}(p_x) = d \sum_{k=0}^{N-1} P_d(k, i_\phi) h(x_d d - kd), \ x_d \in [0 : N - 1]_{\mathbb{Z}}. \tag{2.8.13}$$

2.8.3 Feldkamp Reconstruction Algorithm

Here we present a practical algorithm for 3D cone-beam reconstruction. This is generalized version of 2D fan-beam reconstruction [2, 5, 56, 57] and based on analyzes presented in the work of Feldkamp *et.al.* [20].

The principle of Feldkamp reconstruction algorithm is based on the following assumptions:

- point X-ray source S,

- plane detector,

- reconstructed object is presented by rectangular volume elements "voxels",

- experiment geometry: "source-detector" system is fixed and the object is rotated around the vertical axis inside the cone-beam from source,

- the object is situated completely inside the cone-beam.

For the theoretical purposes it is more efficient to assume existence of a virtual (imaginary) detector, which is placed in the center of reconstructed object parallel to the real detector Figure 2.8. The virtual detector can be obtained using geometrical scaling.

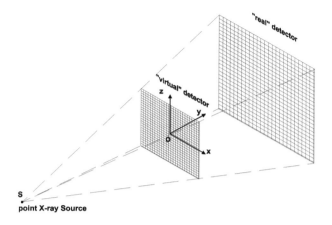

Figure 2.8: Introduction of virtual detector makes description of Feldkamp algorithm more simple.

Consider the geometry of the reconstruction depicted on Figure 2.9. The distance from X-ray source to the point O (center of the object) is $\overline{SO}$. The coordinate system of the reconstructed object is (x,y,z) and it is fixed. The rotated coordinate system is (p,t,z), which is connected to the (x,y,z) in the following way (z axis is the same)

$$\begin{cases} p &= x\cdot\cos(\phi_d)+y\cdot\sin(\phi_d) \\ t &= -x\cdot\sin(\phi_d)+y\cdot\cos(\phi_d). \end{cases} \tag{2.8.14}$$

The coordinate system of the virtual detector is (p,z).

Consider a point A in the object given by the vector $\vec{r}=(x,y,z)$. The ray L goes through this point and hits the virtual detector at the position $[p(\vec{r}),z(\vec{r})]$. A projection of the vector $\vec{r}$ onto the (p,t) plane is the vector $\vec{r}_{tp}$, onto the (t,z) plane is the vector $\vec{r}_{tz}$.

Consider the two triangles SOP and SCA on Figure 2.9(b). These triangles are similar, thus we can write

$$\frac{\overline{SO}}{\overline{SO}+\overline{OC}}=\frac{\overline{OP}}{\overline{CA}} \implies \overline{OP}=\frac{\overline{SO}\cdot\overline{CA}}{\overline{SO}+\overline{OC}}. \tag{2.8.15}$$

Using $\overline{OC}=\vec{r}\cdot\vec{t}$, $\overline{CA}=\vec{r}\cdot\vec{p}$ and $OP=p(\vec{r})$ we obtain the first component of the intersection point

$$p(\vec{r})=\frac{\overline{SO}\cdot(\vec{r}\cdot\vec{p})}{\overline{SO}+\vec{r}\cdot\vec{t}} \tag{2.8.16}$$

35

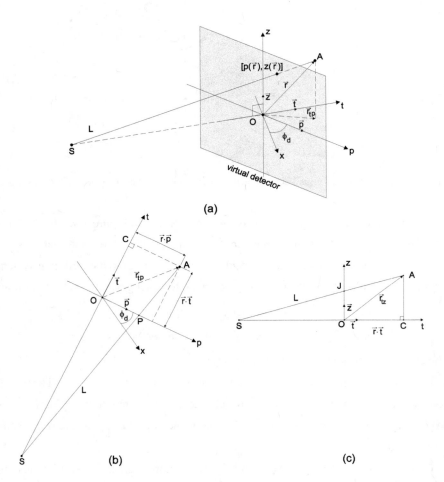

Figure 2.9: Cone-beam reconstruction. X-ray L from source S goes through element of volume $\vec{r}$ (point A) and intersects detector at position $[p(\vec{r}), z(\vec{r})]$. The coordinate system of the virtual detector is (p, z).

36

The triangles on Figure 2.9(c), SOJ and SCA, are also similar, hence

$$\frac{\overline{SO}}{\overline{SO}+\overline{OC}} = \frac{\overline{OJ}}{\overline{CA}} \implies \overline{OJ} = \frac{\overline{SO} \cdot \overline{CA}}{\overline{SO}+\overline{OC}}. \tag{2.8.17}$$

Using $\overline{CA} = \vec{r} \cdot \vec{z}$, $\overline{OC} = \vec{r} \cdot \vec{t}$ and $\overline{OJ} = z(\vec{r})$ we write

$$z(\vec{r}) = \frac{\overline{SO} \cdot (\vec{r} \cdot \vec{z})}{\overline{SO}+\vec{r} \cdot \vec{t}}. \tag{2.8.18}$$

Definition 7. *The function* $P_{3D} : \mathbb{R} \times \mathbb{R} \times [0,2\pi) \rightarrow \mathbb{R}$ *maps the coordinates* (p,z,ϕ_d) *to the values of Radon transform of the density function* $f(x,y,z)$.

The Feldkamp Filtered Backprojection of the $f(x,y,z)$ density reconstruction is expressed as follows[11]

$$f(x,y,z) = \frac{1}{4\pi^2} \int_0^{2\pi} \left\{ \frac{\overline{SO}^2}{(\overline{SO}+\vec{r} \cdot \vec{t})^2} \int_{-\infty}^{\infty} \left[\frac{\overline{SO}}{\sqrt{\overline{SO}^2 + p^2 + z^2}} \cdot P_{3D}(p,z(\vec{r}),\phi_d) \cdot \right. \right.$$
$$\left. \left. \int_{-\infty}^{\infty} |q| e^{2\pi i q(p(\vec{r})-p)} dq \right] dp \right\} d\phi_d \tag{2.8.19}$$

In Equation (2.8.19) the terms

$$\frac{\overline{SO}^2}{(\overline{SO}+\vec{r} \cdot \vec{t})^2} \quad \text{and} \quad \frac{\overline{SO}}{\sqrt{\overline{SO}^2 + p^2 + z^2}} \tag{2.8.20}$$

are weighting coefficients, used to express the contribution of the point A into the projection value $P_{3D}(p,z(\vec{r}),\phi_d)$.

The Feldkamp reconstruction formula (2.8.19) holds only for the circular scanning orbit (X-ray source and detector are fixed and the inspected object rotates without changing its vertical position).

There exist different modifications of the Feldkamp algorithm. Some of them are generalized Feldkamp formulas for different scanning geometries, which can be found in [32, 56, 57]. The error analyzes of the generalized Feldkamp algorithm with variable parameterization of the reconstruction were reported in [58]. This work was supplemental to previous works on the Feldkamp FBP algorithm, and showed (using simulations) that the generalized Feldkamp reconstruction is not sensitive to noise in the input data and allows accurate reconstruction.

---

[11]We present here only the final formula without a proof. The derivations are given in original work [20].

2.8.4 Discrete FBP Algorithm

Let's present the discrete interpretation of the Feldkamp algorithm (2.8.19). In 3D geometry, when detector has N rows with N elements, every detector row is addressed with $y_d \in [0:N-1]_{\mathbb{Z}}$. Thus the coordinates of the sampling points in the detector using (2.8.3) will be

$$\begin{cases} p_x &= (x_d - N/2 + 0.5) \cdot d, \quad x_d \in [0:N-1]_{\mathbb{Z}} \\ z_y &= (y_d - N/2 + 0.5) \cdot d, \quad y_d \in [0:N-1]_{\mathbb{Z}} \end{cases} \tag{2.8.21}$$

where addition of 0.5 shifts the sampling point to the center of the detector element.

Definition 8. *The discrete function*

$$P_{d3D} : [0:N-1]_{\mathbb{Z}} \times [0:N-1]_{\mathbb{Z}} \times [0:\phi_{dmax}-1]_{\mathbb{Z}} \to \mathbb{R}$$

maps (x_d, y_d, i_ϕ) *to the discrete values of the 3D projection* $P_{3D}(p_x, z_y, \phi_{di})$

$$P_{d3D}(x_d, y_d, i_\phi) = P_{3D}(p_x, z_y, \phi_{di}). \tag{2.8.22}$$

Assume that the reconstructed object has a discrete coordinate system (x_O, y_O, z_O) with $x_O \in [0:N-1]_{\mathbb{Z}}$, $y_O \in [0:N-1]_{\mathbb{Z}}$ and $z_O \in [0:N-1]_{\mathbb{Z}}$. The origin O of the reconstructed object has coordinates $(N/2, N/2, N/2)$.

Now we transform the terms of the Equation (2.8.19) to the discrete form setting $\vec{r} = (x_O, y_O, z_O)$ and using

$$\begin{cases} \vec{r} \cdot \vec{p} &= x_O \cdot \cos(\phi_{di}) + y_O \cdot \sin(\phi_{di}) \\ \vec{r} \cdot \vec{t} &= -x_O \cdot \sin(\phi_{di}) + y_O \cdot \cos(\phi_{di}) \\ \vec{r} \cdot \vec{z} &= z_O. \end{cases} \tag{2.8.23}$$

First, using discrete variables, the weighting coefficients are now expressed as

$$\frac{\overline{SO}^2}{(\overline{SO} + \vec{r} \cdot \vec{t})^2} \longrightarrow \frac{\overline{SO}^2}{(\overline{SO} - x_O \cdot \sin(\phi_{di}) + y_O \cdot \cos(\phi_{di}))^2},$$

$$\frac{\overline{SO}}{\sqrt{\overline{SO}^2 + p^2 + z^2}} \longrightarrow \frac{\overline{SO}}{\sqrt{\overline{SO}^2 + p_x^2 + z_y^2}}. \tag{2.8.24}$$

Second, the coordinates of the intersection $[p(\vec{r}), z(\vec{r})]$ are now changed to integral values using the following technique. Let p_d and z_d be the integer discrete functions, that define the integral position of the intersection of the ray L through the voxel (x_O, y_O, z_O) with the detector

$$p_d(x_O, y_O, i_\phi) \in [0 : N-1]_{\mathbb{Z}} \text{ and } z_d(x_O, y_O, z_O, i_\phi) \in [0 : N-1]_{\mathbb{Z}} \ \forall (x_O, y_O, z_O, i_\phi).$$

These functions are expressed now using (2.8.16) and (2.8.18) as

$$\begin{cases} p_d(x_O, y_O, i_\phi) &= \left[\dfrac{\overline{SO} \cdot (x_O \cdot \cos(\phi_{di}) + y_O \cdot \sin(\phi_{di}))}{\overline{SO} - x_O \cdot \sin(\phi_{di}) + y_O \cdot \cos(\phi_{di})} \right]_{int} \\[3mm] z_d(x_O, y_O, z_O, i_\phi) &= \left[\dfrac{\overline{SO} \cdot z_O}{\overline{SO} - x_O \cdot \sin(\phi_{di}) + y_O \cdot \cos(\phi_{di})} \right]_{int} \end{cases} \tag{2.8.25}$$

where the notation $[\cdot]_{int}$ denotes rounding to integer value. Besides simple rounding, some interpolation methods can be used to obtain the right intersection values (p_x, z_y).

Now, using above-defined discrete variables and functions, and the definition of the discrete filtering function (2.8.8), the Feldkamp reconstruction formula can be written as

$$\begin{aligned} f(x_O, y_O, z_O) &= \frac{1}{2\pi\phi_{dmax}} \sum_{i_\phi=0}^{\phi_{dmax}-1} \Bigg\{ \frac{\overline{SO}^2 \cdot d}{(\overline{SO} - x_O \cdot \sin(\phi_{di}) + y_O \cdot \cos(\phi_{di}))^2} \cdot \\ &\quad \sum_{x_d=0}^{N-1} \Big(\frac{\overline{SO}}{\sqrt{\overline{SO}^2 + p_x^2 + z_y^2}} P_{d3D}(x_d, z_d(x_O, y_O, z_O, i_\phi), i_\phi) \cdot \\ &\quad h(p_d(x_O, y_O, i_\phi) d - x_d d) \Big) \Bigg\}. \end{aligned} \tag{2.8.26}$$

Defining the filtering function $W_{d3D}(x_O, y_O, z_O, i_\phi)$ as

$$\begin{aligned} W_{d3D}(x_O, y_O, z_O, i_\phi) &= d \sum_{x_d=0}^{N-1} P_{d3D}(x_d, z_d(x_O, y_O, z_O, i_\phi), i_\phi) \cdot \\ &\quad h(p_d(x_O, y_O, i_\phi) d - x_d d) \frac{\overline{SO}}{\sqrt{\overline{SO}^2 + p_x^2 + z_y^2}} \end{aligned} \tag{2.8.27}$$

we rewrite the continuous Equation (2.8.26) in discrete form

$$f(x_O, y_O, z_O) = \frac{1}{2\pi\phi_{dmax}} \sum_{i_\phi=0}^{\phi_{dmax}-1} \frac{\overline{SO}^2 \cdot W_{d3D}(x_O, y_O, z_O, i_\phi)}{(\overline{SO} - x_O \cdot \sin(\phi_{di}) + y_O \cdot \cos(\phi_{di}))^2}. \tag{2.8.28}$$

As the number of voxels in the reconstructed object is N^3 and for the real experiment the number of projections $\phi_{d\,max}$ is in $O(N)$, the computational complexity of the Filtered Backprojection algorithm is $O(N^4)$. The most computationally extensive step in FBP is the backprojection, which must be performed for every voxel in the object for every projection. As it will be shown in the next parts, the modifications of this algorithm make it possible to speed-up the backprojection step.

2.9 Conclusion

In this chapter we introduced the definitions and derived the formulas for the Radon transform and for the reconstruction from projections. The overview of the reconstruction algorithms gives comprehension of the reconstruction techniques. For the different cases of reconstruction and application-specific features refer to above-mentioned literature. Filtered Backprojection was chosen as the primary method for the reconstruction from projections. This method gives good reconstruction results especially applying to non-destructive testing, despite the high computational complexity. In section 2.8.4 the discrete version of the Feldkamp reconstruction algorithm was presented. This algorithm will be used as basis for the practical algorithm, which will be introduced in the next section.

Chapter 3

Rapid Practical Reconstruction

The reconstruction from projections has a lot of scientific applications. The constant expansion of the tomographic applications leads to the continual improvement of the reconstruction algorithms and practical scanning methods. There are two main application fields of the CT: medical applications and non-destructive testing (NDT). For both fields the problem of rapid reconstruction is one of the most actual.

The clinical applications actively use the tomography and it became one of the most important tools in the modern diagnostics. This application field differs greatly from NDT. Positron Emission Tomography (PET) and Single Photon Emission Tomography (SPECT) are applied in the clinical diagnostics [59]. PET and SPECT use different methods for the reconstruction from projections including Fourier and FBP reconstruction algorithms.

The NDT requires practical CT reconstruction methods for the material testing [6, 60, 61] where the CT can be seen as nondestructive microscopy, delivering cross sections. CT technique provides testing of all kinds of materials and product control: welding joints, flaw detection, density change, etc. Here, the FBP method suits for the big class of problems, providing the fast and appropriate reconstruction results.

For higher profitability of the 3D CT technique in practical NDT applications the reconstruction methods with the following features are required:

- an algorithm with reduction of artifacts and noise in the reconstructed image,

- small numerical costs of the reconstruction for a fast result output,

- the reconstruction should be done during the projections measurements,

- the reconstruction time must be smaller or comparable with CT experiment time in order to visualize the results of the density reconstruction at the end of the measurements.

The improvement of the current CT technique for NDT field can be done in the following way:

- search for the modification of the FBP reconstruction algorithm in order to decrease the reconstruction time,

- accelerate the implementation of the existing algorithm using the parallel processing technique,

- apply custom hardware design, that performs the reconstruction using FBP algorithm.

In this chapter we discuss the modification of the FBP algorithm for 3D cone-beam projections. This is a practical algorithm, that speed-up the reconstruction significantly. In section 3.2 the related work in the field of parallel processing will be described.

3.1 Cylindrical Algorithm

The analyses of the reconstruction algorithms and the practical experience in applications point out the Feldkamp FBP algorithm, that gives the best results of the reconstruction in the NDT applications. The Equation (2.8.28), presented in the previous chapter, can be directly implemented on a PC (Algorithm 1).

Our goal is to find the fast implementation of the FBP algorithm, applied to the NDT field. The necessity of the modification and optimization of Algorithm 1 is based on the fact, that the straightforward implementation of this algorithm for the real application is slow:

Algorithm 1 Feldkamp Reconstruction Algorithm

---
initialize the 3D density volume
for projection $i_\phi = 0$ to $\phi_{d\,max} - 1$ **do**
  for all voxels (x_O, y_O, z_O) **do**
    calculate $p_d(x_O, y_O, i_\phi)$ and $z_d(x_O, y_O, z_O, i_\phi)$ (*Equation (2.8.25)*)
    calculate $W_{d3D}(x_O, y_O, z_O, i_\phi)$ (*Equation (2.8.27)*)
    backproject the value $W_{d3D}(x_O, y_O, z_O, i_\phi)$ (*Equation (2.8.28)*)
  end for
end for

- the rotation of the whole reconstructed volume by the angle $\phi_{d\,i}$ is a highly time consuming operation,

- all coordinates of the ray-detector intersection ((2.8.16), (2.8.18)) and weighting coefficients (2.8.20) must be calculated for all voxels for each projection angle.

All these operations are performed using floating-point arithmetic. Thus, for the rapid implementation on PC and in hardware, the number of complex operations (e.g. using floating-point numbers), performed for one voxel during the backprojection, must be minimized. The method, that allows the minimization of floating-point calculations in the Feldkamp FBP algorithm, was proposed in Fraunhofer Institute for non-destructive testing[1] and was described in Buck's PhD thesis [61]. The Buck's suggestion was to use the cylindrical coordinates in the Feldkamp algorithm for the reconstruction from the cone-beam projections. This allows to simplify the calculations and to compute all parameters for the reconstruction (weighting coefficients, coordinates of the ray-detector intersection) only once, for the rotation angle equal to $0°$, and store them in tables. The cylindrical coordinates allow to operate with the reconstruction volume without use of transcendental functions and multiplication operations.

There are several tables that are used in the modified algorithm:

- the Volume Table,

---
[1] Fraunhofer Institut für Zerstörungsfreie Prüfverfahren (IZFP), Saarbrücken [62]

- the Geometry Table,

- the Weighting Coefficients Table,

- the Filtered Projections Table.

In this section the construction of these tables will be described, and they will be used in the modified FBP algorithm.

3.1.1 Reconstruction Coordinate System

During the reconstruction process the Cartesian grid of the object is rotated around the z-axis going from projection i_ϕ to $i_\phi + 1$. Normally this (2.8.23) is done using two steps:

1. obtain the values of the transcendental functions with the discrete angle ϕ_{di} of a projection as an argument, and

2. multiply these values with the x_O and y_O values of the Cartesian coordinates.

In this case, to speed-up the rotation, the polar coordinates are preferable.

The FBP using the cylindrical grid does not introduce the artifacts in the reconstructed image, as e.g. the Fourier reconstruction method. In the Fourier reconstruction the experiment data is interpolated from the polar grid to the Cartesian and this results in the artifacts in the final image (section 2.5.1). Apart this, the Fourier reconstruction method cannot be directly applied to the reconstruction from the cone-beam projections[2]. In the cylindrical algorithm the final reconstructed density, placed on the cylindrical grid, can be interpolated to the Cartesian grid with sufficiently small errors.

We introduce the *continuous* cylindrical coordinates $(z_{Oa}, r_{Oa}, \phi_{Oa})$ for the reconstruction object. The whole volume is divided into discrete elements – *voxels*. The cylindrical volume has the following parameters of the voxel distribution[3]:

- z_{Omax} is the maximal number of planes in the volume,

---

[2] only using "rebinning" technique [5]
[3] see section 3.1.7 for the formal definitions

- r_{Omax} is the maximal number of radial elements (circles) in one plane,

- ϕ_{Omax} is the maximal number of voxels, placed on a radial element in a plane,

and the following counters:

- planes counter $z_O \in [0 : z_{Omax} - 1]_{\mathbb{Z}}$

- radial elements counter $r_O \in [0 : r_{Omax} - 1]_{\mathbb{Z}}$

- angle counter $\phi_O \in [0 : \phi_{Omax} - 1]_{\mathbb{Z}}$.

With this notation the voxel A can be addressed with the discrete indices (z_O, r_O, ϕ_O), which are used to access the values in tables, corresponding to this element A.

3.1.2 Distribution of Voxels

Let's discuss the parameters of the voxel distribution. If the detector row has N elements, then the region that can be reconstructed is not more than $N \times N$ (Cartesian grid) [5, 27]. This is due to the geometry resolution of the detector. All our derivations and conclusions about the distribution will use the fact that the number N is sufficiently large, e.g. more than 256 for the real applications. The number of projections is always at most N, the increase provides the better quality of the reconstruction image, but does not change the geometrical resolution. For our discussions we assume $\phi_{dmax} \leq N$.

In spite of the notable speed-up of the backprojection with cylindrical coordinates [61, 63], there is one drawback, namely the polar and, accordingly, cylindrical grid does not coincide with the Cartesian grid, and one can note that the voxels, situated along the inner radial elements, are smaller than those along outer radial elements (Figure 3.1(a)). For the best reconstructed picture quality one needs to distribute the voxels with uniform density. At first, we set the maximum number of radial elements to $N/2$.

Second, as we rotate the cylindrical grid the number of voxels placed on a radial element must be connected to the number of projections, i.e. rotations of the object. This is used in cyclic addressing of the reconstruction grid. Thus, the special

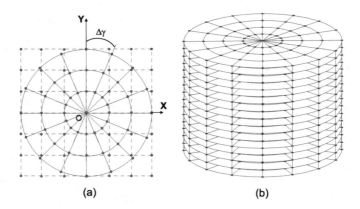

Figure 3.1: Radial distribution of voxels in the reconstructed object. (a) – in-plane voxel distribution, (b) – object, represented as set of planes in cylindrical coordinates.

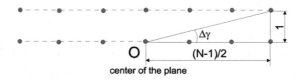

Figure 3.2: $\Delta\gamma$ is the smallest radial step for the polar grid.

integrality condition, that defines the correspondence of the ϕ_{Omax} to the number of projections ϕ_{dmax} must be preserved.

Condition 1. *The ratio ϕ_{Omax}/ϕ_{dmax} for $\phi_{Omax} \geq \phi_{dmax}$ (and ϕ_{dmax}/ϕ_{Omax} otherwise) must be integral.*

The smallest angle between two neighbor voxels on a radial element (Figure 3.2) can be obtained as

$$\Delta\gamma = arctan(\frac{2}{N-1}), \qquad (3.1.1)$$

so the number of voxels on one radial element r_O is $\phi_{Omax} \approx \lceil 2\pi/\Delta\gamma \rceil$.

There are two possibilities of the in-plane pixel distribution on the polar grid:

1. number ϕ_{Omax} is equal for each radial element r_O, and

2. number ϕ_{Omax} is dependent on the radius of the element r_O.

The first distribution leads to the oversampling in center of the polar grid. The number of pixels on every radial element in this case is for $n_\phi \in \mathbb{Z}_{\geq 1}$

$$\begin{cases} \phi_{Omax} = n_\phi \cdot \phi_{dmax} & \text{if } \phi_{Omax} \geq \phi_{dmax} \\ \phi_{dmax} = n_\phi \cdot \phi_{Omax} & \text{if } \phi_{Omax} < \phi_{dmax}. \end{cases} \qquad (3.1.2)$$

The second type of pixel distribution has variable value of ϕ_{Omax} for each radial element. By $\phi_{Omax}(i)$ with $i \in [0 : r_{Omax} - 1]_\mathbb{Z}$ we denote the array of ϕ_{Omax} values. Algorithm 2 presents the calculation of the variable number of pixels $\phi_{Omax}()$, which is a modified version of the similar algorithm proposed in [64]. For this case the ratio between the values $\phi_{Omax}(i)$ and ϕ_{dmax} will be defined for the $n_\phi(i) \in \mathbb{Z} \ \forall i$ as

$$\begin{cases} \phi_{Omax}(i) = n_\phi(i) \cdot \phi_{dmax} & \text{if } \phi_{Omax}(i) \geq \phi_{dmax} \\ \phi_{dmax} = n_\phi(i) \cdot \phi_{Omax}(i) & \text{if } \phi_{Omax}(i) < \phi_{dmax}. \end{cases} \qquad (3.1.3)$$

Algorithm 2 Calculation of the Variable ϕ_{Omax}

---

initialize $\phi_{Omax}()$

$\phi_{Omax}(0) \leftarrow 1$ *(center pixel of the plane)*

for $i = 1$ to $r_{Omax} - 1$ **do**

     $\phi_{Omax}(i) \leftarrow \lceil 2 \cdot \pi \cdot (i - 0.5) \rceil$ *(initial $\phi_{Omax}(i)$)*

     if $\phi_{Omax}(i) \neq \phi_{dmax}$ **then**

         if $\phi_{Omax}(i) > \phi_{dmax}$ **then**

             increase $\phi_{Omax}(i)$ until the Condition 1 holds for $\phi_{Omax}(i) > \phi_{dmax}$

         else

             increase $\phi_{Omax}(i)$ until the Condition 1 holds for $\phi_{dmax} > \phi_{Omax}(i)$

         end if

     end if

end for

For example, in real applications we use $N = 512$ and $\phi_{dmax} = 400$. Using this we obtain:

- The Cartesian grid has $N^2 = 262144$ voxels in one plane.

- The cylindrical grid with constant number of voxels using (3.1.1) has $\phi_{Omax} = 1600$ and $r_{Omax} = 256$, the total number of voxels in one plane is 409600.

- The cylindrical grid with variable number of voxels (Algorithm 2) has

$$\phi_{Omax}() \in \{4, \dots, 1600\}, \quad r_{Omax} = 256$$

and the total number of voxels in one plane is 208535.

This example shows that the introduction of the cylindrical grid leads to the increase of the number of reconstructed voxels. Some of the practical implementations that use polar coordinates [61, 64], have two cases:

1. the variable voxel distribution with the total number of voxels comparable to N^2,

2. the constant number of voxels but reducing the number of voxels on each radial element.

For example, the coefficient n_ϕ from (3.1.2) for the second case can be "2" or "3". This gives the number of voxels almost the same as in Cartesian grid, and preserves the reconstructed image quality, admissible for the NDT applications.

Now and for the future we use for description the constant number of voxels $\phi_{Omax} > \phi_{dmax}$ and

$$n_\phi = \phi_{Omax}/\phi_{dmax} = 2.$$

This is done for the simplicity of the description and suits for the NDT practical applications. All the formulas, e.g. for the Geometry Table in section 3.1.7, can be converted without additional effort to the case with variable number of voxels. Finally, the maximum number of planes that can be reconstructed will be defined in section 3.1.7.

3.1.3 Rotation of the Cylindrical Grid

As it was mentioned before, the cylindrical grid gives the best solution to the rotation of the object. Here we state and prove the Lemma about the cyclical addressing of the elements placed on the polar grid using the *modulo computation*

$$y > x \pmod{y} \geq 0.$$

We subtract the projection number i_ϕ (recall (2.8.1)) multiplied by $n_\phi \in \mathbb{Z}_{\geq 1}$ from the address of the voxel, placed on a radial element in a plane and obtain the new address using modulo ϕ_{Omax}. The following Lemma holds for our assumption of the constant number of voxels $\phi_{Omax} > \phi_{dmax}$.

Lemma 1. *The pixels on a radial element can be cyclically addressed using the argument* $\left[\phi_O - n_\phi \cdot i_\phi\right]$ *(mod* ϕ_{Omax}*) with* $n_\phi = \phi_{Omax}/\phi_{dmax}$.

Proof. Consider the 2D CT experiment. Let ψ_d be an angle of the object rotation and the direction of the rotation is counter-clockwise. The coordinate system of the object is polar (r_{Oa}, ϕ_{Oa}).

In *position 2* on Figure 3.3 the ray L goes from the source through the pixel A' with coordinates (r_{Oa}, ϕ_{Oa}) and hits the detector at P'. Now, if we consider *position 1*, the same ray L goes through the point A with coordinates $(r_{Oa}, \phi_{Oa} - \psi_d)$ and intersects with the detector at point P. Symmetry gives $P = P'$. The angle ψ_d is expressed in discrete form as $n_\phi \cdot i_\phi$ with integer $n_\phi = \phi_{Omax}/\phi_{dmax}$ and we obtain the discrete coordinates of the point A

$$(r_O, \left[\phi_O - n_\phi \cdot i_\phi\right] \ (\text{mod} \ \phi_{Omax})),$$

Thus, in order to rotate the polar grid, the modulo computation can be used applied to the integer counters. This avoids the use of transcendental functions for the rotation. □

3.1.4 Significant Parameters of the Experiment

The practical algorithm for CT deals with the restrictions, which are determined by the real experiment. We do not discuss e.g. beam-hardening and other physical effects [2, 5] that influence the CT experiment. The goal is to take into account the limitations of the geometry, e.g. physical sizes of the objects, the region that can be reconstructed from projections, the magnification of the object.

In order to determine the region between the source and the detector that can be reconstructed from the projections, we present the information about the characteristics of the practical CT experiment geometry:

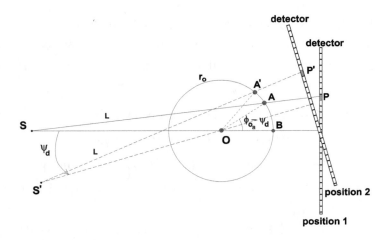

Figure 3.3: Rotation of the X-ray source - detector system by an angle ψ_d.

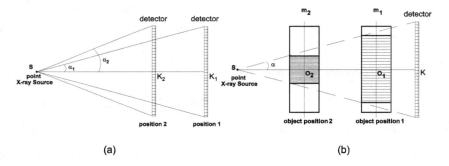

(a)   (b)

Figure 3.4: Description of the half-beam opening angle (a) and the magnification factor (b).

- the half-beam opening angle α,

- the magnification factor m,

- the physical size of the detector element d.

Currently, most of the CT systems use cone-beam X-ray sources and the half-beam opening angle for CT experiment is controlled by the distance X-ray source - detector. The geometries with different source - detector distances are depicted on Figure 3.4(a). Moving the detector closer to the X-ray source S increases the half-beam opening angle.

50

The magnification factor m characterizes the enlargement of the part of the reconstructed object or the magnification of a small object. Changing the position of the inspected object between the source and the detector alters the value of the magnification factor. For example, showed on Figure 3.4(b) for a constant angle α we have

$$m_1 = \overline{SK}/\overline{SO_1} \quad m_2 = \overline{SK}/\overline{SO_2} \quad m_2 > m_1.$$

The physical size of the detector element (pixel) is used in geometry calculations and defines the resolution of the detector. As it was mentioned before we assume the square detector with $N \times N$ pixels. These detector pixels have physical size $d \times d$, where d is a distance between the centers of the two adjacent pixels. As in section 2.8.1 the detector pixels are situated close together. In practice there can be different modifications of the detectors [65]. The parameters of these detectors must be included into the calculations, e.g. length and width of the non-square pixels.

3.1.5 Volume Table

The density function of the reconstructed object (volume) is presented as a table used in the backprojection. This table is addressed cyclically during the reconstruction, and at the end of this process consists of the reconstructed density data.

Definition 9. *By $V_c[z_O, r_O, \phi_O]$ we denote the table*

$$V_c : [0 : z_{Omax} - 1]_{\mathbb{Z}} \times [0 : r_{Omax} - 1]_{\mathbb{Z}} \times [0 : \phi_{Omax} - 1]_{\mathbb{Z}} \rightarrow \mathbb{R}$$

that maps the discrete coordinates of the voxel (z_O, r_O, ϕ_O) to the backprojected values.

The final result, that is located in the Volume Table $V_c[\ ]$ can be interpolated to the Cartesian grid using linear interpolation [66] or Near-Exact interpolation [67]. This is necessary for the standard visualization of the reconstructed image, but the visualization can be performed also directly in the cylindrical coordinates. This is dependent on the particular application of the CT. In this work we do not consider interpolation to the Cartesian grid.

3.1.6 Filtered Projection Table

In section 2.8.2 we showed that the projections from the detector must be filtered through the convolution (2.8.13) using special Ramp filter function, e.g. (2.8.10).

The backprojection requires the projection value addressed with ray-detector intersection coordinates $[p(\vec{r}), z(\vec{r})]$ given by (2.8.16) and (2.8.18). This projection value is filtered and then backprojected. Hence, in order to reconstruct the whole volume all the projection values are accessed and filtered. Thus, the equivalent substitution will be:

- filter projection data,

- store filtered data in the table,

- access this table during the reconstruction.

The experiment projection data, denoted by $P_{d3D}(x_d, y_d, i_\phi)$ for a projection i_ϕ, is filtered line by line y_d and stored for the further use. Here we use the definition of the p_x and z_y given by (2.8.21).

Definition 10. *By* $FD[x_d, y_d, i_\phi]$ *we denote the table*

$$FD : [0 : N-1]_{\mathbb{Z}} \times [0 : N-1]_{\mathbb{Z}} \times [0 : \phi_{dmax} - 1]_{\mathbb{Z}} \to \mathbb{R}$$

that maps the discrete coordinate of the square detector for a projection i_ϕ *to the filtered projection data as*

$$FD[x_d, y_d, i_\phi] = d \sum_{k=0}^{N-1} P_{d3D}(k, y_d, i_\phi) h(x_d \cdot d - k \cdot d) \frac{\overline{SO}}{\sqrt{\overline{SO}^2 + p_x^2 + z_y^2}} \quad \forall \, x_d, y_d, i_\phi.$$

$$(3.1.4)$$

By $FD[*, y_d, i_\phi]$ we denote a row y_d in a projection i_ϕ; by $FD[*, y_d, *]$ we denote one row y_d for all filtered projections. The filtering of a projection i_ϕ is presented in Algorithm 3.

Algorithm 3 Filtering of a Projection

---

    initialize $FD[*,*,i_\phi]$

    for detector row $y_d = 0$ to $N-1$ **do**

        for element in a row $x_d = 0$ to $N-1$ **do**

            $FD[x_d,y_d,i_\phi] \leftarrow d\sum_{k=0}^{N-1} P_{d3D}(k,y_d,i_\phi)h(x_d \cdot d - k \cdot d)\dfrac{\overline{SO}}{\sqrt{\overline{SO}^2+p_x^2+z_y^2}}$

        end for

    end for

3.1.7 Geometry Table

The time consuming part during the backprojection is the determination of the ray-detector intersection (2.8.25) for each voxel for each projection. These intersection points can be calculated before the backprojection, because they are defined by the geometry of the experiment, but are independent from the properties of the reconstructed object. The address of the detector pixel is stored as an absolute detector address which is expressed as $z_d \cdot N + p_d$.

Definition 11. *By $INS[z_O,r_O,\phi_O]$ we denote the table*

$$INS: [0:z_{Omax}-1]_\mathbb{Z} \times [0:r_{Omax}-1]_\mathbb{Z} \times [0:\phi_{Omax}-1]_\mathbb{Z} \to \mathbb{Z}$$

that maps the coordinates of a voxel onto the absolute detector address of the ray-detector intersection

$$INS[z_O,r_O,\phi_O] = z_d \cdot N + p_d.$$

The Geometry Table has the same dimensions as the Volume Table, because we define the intersection point for every voxel. This is enough for the reconstruction from the projections and the table is addressed cyclically together with the Volume and the Weighting Coefficients Tables using Lemma 1. This is described later in section 3.1.9.

In order to calculate the Geometry Table for the whole volume, we need to obtain two coordinates of the ray-detector intersection (2.8.25) for each voxel:

- horizontal intersection coordinate p_d, and

- vertical intersection coordinate z_d.

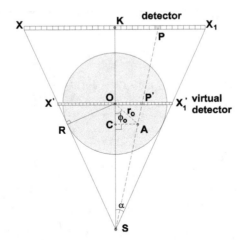

Figure 3.5: Calculation of the horizontal intersection coordinate. Only the points that are inside the circular region can be accessed.

Horizontal Intersection Coordinate

To obtain the horizontal intersection coordinate p_d we discuss the geometry of the plane that is situated in the center of the object. We call this plane *a central plane*. For each pixel in this plane we consider a ray, that goes from the X-ray source through the center of the pixel and hits the detector (2.8.16). Figure 3.5 shows the geometry of the experiment for the central plane. Let XX_1 be a detector row, that lies in the same horizontal plane as the X-ray source. Usually[4], this is a row with the vertical coordinate $y_d = N/2$.

The distance $\overline{OR}$ on Figure 3.5 is the maximal radius R_{max} of the reconstruction, i.e. all points, that are inside the circular region with R_{max}, can be reconstructed from the projections. We obtain this value using known parameters of the CT geometry. If $\overline{KX_1} = d \cdot N/2$ is one half of the detector, then using two triangles SOR and SKX_1 and magnification factor m we have

---

[4]special turning of the X-ray tube and detector positions

$$R_{max} = \overline{OR} = \overline{SO} \cdot \sin(\alpha)$$
$$= \frac{\overline{SK}}{m} \cdot \frac{\overline{KX_1}}{\overline{SX_1}}$$
$$= \frac{\overline{SK}}{\overline{SX_1}} \cdot \frac{\overline{KX_1}}{m}$$
$$= \frac{\cos(\alpha)}{m} \cdot \overline{KX_1}$$
$$= \frac{N \cdot d}{2 \cdot m} \cdot \cos(\alpha). \tag{3.1.5}$$

Using R_{max} we can define now the distance Δr_O between the centers of two adjacent pixels and the physical distance from the origin of a plane to the radial element r_O

$$r_{Oa} = r_O \cdot \Delta r_O, \quad \Delta r_O = \frac{2R_{max}}{2r_{Omax} - 1}, \quad r_O \in [0 : r_{Omax} - 1]_{\mathbb{Z}}. \tag{3.1.6}$$

By analogy with (2.8.1) we define the radial interval for the pixels on a radial element. Using ϕ_O as a counter we obtain

$$\phi_{Oa} = \phi_O \cdot \Delta\phi_O, \quad \Delta\phi_O = \frac{2\pi}{\phi_{Omax}}, \quad \phi_O \in [0 : \phi_{Omax} - 1]_{\mathbb{Z}}. \tag{3.1.7}$$

Using discrete coordinates of the pixel A (r_O, ϕ_O) and taking the triangle SCA we obtain the following:

$$\overline{OA} = r_{Oa}$$
$$\overline{CA} = r_{Oa} \cdot \sin(\phi_{Oa})$$
$$\overline{SC} = \overline{SO} - r_{Oa} \cdot \cos(\phi_{Oa}). \tag{3.1.8}$$

Consider two triangles SCA and SOP'. As these triangles are similar, we write

$$\overline{OP'} = \frac{\overline{SO} \cdot \overline{CA}}{\overline{SC}} = \frac{\overline{SO} \cdot r_{Oa} \cdot \sin(\phi_{Oa})}{\overline{SO} - r_{Oa} \cdot \cos(\phi_{Oa})}. \tag{3.1.9}$$

The ray from the X-ray source S goes through the pixel A and hits the detector at the point P

$$\overline{KP} = \overline{OP'} \cdot m = \frac{\overline{SO} \cdot m \cdot r_{Oa} \cdot \sin(\phi_{Oa})}{\overline{SO} - r_{Oa} \cdot \cos(\phi_{Oa})}. \tag{3.1.10}$$

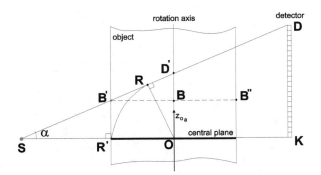

Figure 3.6: 3D reconstruction geometry. $\overline{OB}$ – half of the reconstruction height, $\overline{KD}$ consists of $N/2$ detector rows.

Thus we obtained the intersect point of a ray for the pixel A in the central plane. Using

$$\overline{XP} = \overline{KP} + (\frac{N}{2} - 1) \cdot d$$

we write the integral horizontal coordinate

$$p_d = \frac{1}{d} \cdot \frac{\overline{SO} \cdot m \cdot r_{Oa} \cdot \sin(\phi_{Oa})}{\overline{SO} - r_{Oa} \cdot \cos(\phi_{Oa})} + \frac{N}{2} - 1. \qquad (3.1.11)$$

All horizontal intersect points are centered with the term $(N/2 - 1)$, because the detector elements in the detector row are counted in the detector row from X to X_1 (from 0 to $N - 1$).

Absolute Intersection Coordinate

Before we obtain the calculations for the Geometry Table we need to determine how many planes can be reconstructed using the restrictions of the experiment geometry. The total number of planes z_{Omax} is less than the number of detector rows N and depends on the experiment geometry.

Consider Figure 3.6 where we take only the upper part of the object, counting from the central plane. We need to find the part of the volume, which is completely covered with X-ray radiation. This part can be reconstructed from the projections.

For example, the part of the object with the height $\overline{BD'}$ can not be reconstructed, because some part of the projections information is missing [27].

The height $\overline{OB}$ of the reconstruction cylinder can be obtained as follows (using similar triangles $SR'B'$ and SOD')

$$\begin{aligned}
\overline{OB} = \overline{R'B'} &= \overline{OD'} \cdot \frac{\overline{SR'}}{\overline{SO}} \\
&= \overline{OD'} \cdot \frac{\overline{SO} - \overline{OR'}}{\overline{SO}} \\
&= \overline{OD'} \cdot (1 - \frac{\overline{OR'}}{\overline{SO}}).
\end{aligned}$$

In the triangle SOR the distance $\overline{OR'}$ is equal to $\overline{SO} \cdot \sin(\alpha)$. Thus

$$\begin{aligned}
\overline{OB} &= \overline{OD'} \cdot (1 - \frac{\overline{SO} \cdot \sin(\alpha)}{\overline{SO}}) \\
&= \overline{OD'} \cdot (1 - \sin(\alpha)). \quad (3.1.12)
\end{aligned}$$

The part of the detector $\overline{KD}$ is equal to $N \cdot d/2$ and $\overline{OD'} = \overline{KD}/m = N \cdot d/(2m)$. Using that the height $\overline{OB}$ is only the half of the reconstruction cylinder height Z_h we obtain this value

$$Z_h = 2 \cdot \overline{OB} = \frac{N \cdot d}{m} \cdot (1 - \sin(\alpha)). \quad (3.1.13)$$

For the reconstruction volume we want to have almost cubic voxels. Thus we need that the height and the width of the voxel must be equal. Hence

$$\Delta z_O = \Delta r_O, \quad z_{Oa} = z_O \cdot \Delta z_O. \quad (3.1.14)$$

The interval Z_h has z_{Omax} planes with height Δz_O, thus

$$z_{Omax} = \frac{Z_h}{\Delta z_O} = \frac{N \cdot d}{m \cdot \Delta r_O} \cdot (1 - \sin(\alpha)). \quad (3.1.15)$$

Figure 3.7 depicts the geometry of a non-central plane with the vertical coordinate z_{Oa}. The ray L from the source S goes through the voxel A_O with the coordinates $(z_{Oa}, r_{Oa}, \phi_{Oa})$ and hits the pixel P_O of the detector. Using the geometry similar to the central plane (3.1.8)-(3.1.11) we obtain the vertical intersection coordinate

$$z_d = \frac{1}{d} \cdot \frac{\overline{SO} \cdot m \cdot (z_O - z_{Omax}/2) \cdot \Delta z_O}{\overline{SO} - r_{Oa} \cdot \cos(\phi_{Oa})} + \frac{N}{2} - 1. \quad (3.1.16)$$

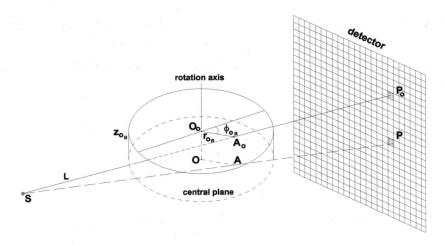

Figure 3.7: Obtaining the vertical ray L - detector intersection coordinate.

The planes are counted from the upper face of the reconstructed volume and the central plane will be $z_{Omax}/2 - 1$. There is a term $z_O - z_{Omax}/2$ that aligns the plane relative to the center of the reconstruction volume. The term $N/2 - 1$ is used for the same purpose. The plane $z_O = 0$ access detector rows counting from the upper detector row, whereas the central plane access the row with coordinate $y_d = N/2 - 1$.

Now, using two coordinates p_d (3.1.11) and z_d (3.1.16), we can write the absolute detector address of the ray-detector intersection

$$
\begin{aligned}
INS[z_O, r_O, \phi_O] &= z_d \cdot N + p_d \\
&= \frac{1}{d} \cdot \frac{\overline{SO} \cdot N \cdot m \cdot (z_O - z_{Omax}/2) \cdot \Delta z_O}{\overline{SO} - r_{Oa} \cdot \cos(\phi_{Oa})} \\
&+ \frac{1}{d} \cdot \frac{\overline{SO} \cdot m \cdot r_{Oa} \cdot \sin(\phi_{Oa})}{\overline{SO} - r_{Oa} \cdot \cos(\phi_{Oa})} \\
&+ N \cdot (\frac{N}{2} - 1) + \frac{N}{2} - 1.
\end{aligned}
\tag{3.1.17}
$$

Algorithm 4 provides the calculation of the geometry matrix.

Algorithm 4 Calculation of the Geometry Table
---
initialize $INS[\ ]$

$R_{max} \leftarrow \cos(\alpha) \cdot N \cdot d/(2m)$ *(the region of the reconstruction)*

$\Delta r_O \leftarrow 2R_{max}/(2r_{Omax} - 1)$ *(size of the voxel)*

$z_{Omax} \leftarrow \frac{N \cdot d}{m \cdot \Delta r_O} \cdot (1 - \sin(\alpha))$ *(the maximal number of planes)*

for plane $z_O = 0$ to $z_{Omax} - 1$ **do**

    for $r_O = 0$ to $r_{Omax} - 1$ **do**

        for $\phi_O = 0$ to $\phi_{Omax} - 1$ **do**

            $p_d \leftarrow \frac{1}{d} \cdot \frac{\overline{SO} \cdot m \cdot r_{Oa} \cdot \sin(\phi_{Oa})}{\overline{SO} - r_{Oa} \cdot \cos(\phi_{Oa})} + \frac{N}{2} - 1$ *(the horizontal coordinate)*

            $z_d \leftarrow \frac{\overline{SO} \cdot m \cdot (z_O - z_{Omax}/2) \cdot \Delta z_O}{\overline{SO} - r_{Oa} \cdot \cos(\phi_{Oa})} + \frac{N}{2} - 1$ *(the vertical coordinate)*

            $INS[z_O, r_O, \phi_O] \leftarrow z_d \cdot N + p_d$ *(store the absolute address)*

        end for

    end for

end for

3.1.8 Weighting Coefficients Table

In this section we discuss the computation of the weighting coefficients. Equation (2.8.24) gives the discrete form of the weighting coefficients, that must be calculated for every voxel during the reconstruction.

The weighting coefficient

$$\frac{\overline{SO}}{\sqrt{\overline{SO}^2 + p^2 + z^2}}$$

is used during the filter operation described by Algorithm 3. This coefficient is not stored, because it is a part of the calculation of the Filtered Projection Table.

We represent another weighting coefficient from (2.8.24) in polar coordinates. Consider Figure 3.8. The polar axis coincides with the Y-axis in XY-plane and has an opposite direction[5]. The transformation from one coordinate system into another

---

[5]This direction of the polar axis was selected in order to comply with the Buck's implementation of the Cylindrical Algorithm [61]. Any other directions in XY-plane are possible, but the translation (3.1.18) between the polar and Cartesian coordinates systems must be modified.

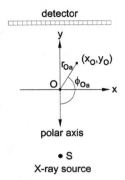

detector

polar axis

• S
X-ray source

Figure 3.8: Two reconstruction coordinate systems, Cartesian and polar.

is expressed as:

$$\begin{cases} r_{Oa} = \sqrt{x_O^2 + y_O^2} \\ \phi_{Oa} = \frac{\pi}{2} + \text{atan}\frac{y_O}{x_O} \end{cases} \quad \text{and} \quad \begin{cases} x_O = r_{Oa} \cdot \cos(\phi_{Oa} - \frac{\pi}{2}) = r_{Oa} \cdot \sin(\phi_{Oa}) \\ y_O = r_{Oa} \cdot \sin(\phi_{Oa} - \frac{\pi}{2}) = -r_{Oa} \cdot \cos(\phi_{Oa}) \end{cases}$$
$$(3.1.18)$$

We plug the formulas for x_O and y_O into (2.8.24).

$$\frac{\overline{SO}^2}{(\overline{SO} - x_O \cdot \sin(\phi_{di}) + y_O \cdot \cos(\phi_{di}))^2} =$$
$$\frac{\overline{SO}^2}{(\overline{SO} - r_{Oa} \cdot \sin(\phi_{Oa}) \cdot \sin(\phi_{di}) - r_{Oa} \cdot \cos(\phi_{Oa}) \cdot \cos(\phi_{di}))^2} =$$
$$\frac{\overline{SO}^2}{(\overline{SO} - r_{Oa} \cdot \cos(\phi_{Oa} + \phi_{di}))^2}$$

Recall that $\phi_{Omax} = n_\phi \cdot \phi_{dmax}$. Using $\Delta\phi_{di} = n_\phi \cdot \Delta\phi_O$, the sum of the discrete angles $(\phi_{Oa} + \phi_{di})$ can be expressed as

$$\begin{aligned} \phi_a' &= \phi_O \cdot \Delta\phi_O + i_\phi \cdot \Delta\phi_{di} \\ &= \phi_O \cdot \Delta\phi_O + i_\phi \cdot n_\phi \cdot \Delta\phi_O \\ &= \left[(\phi_O + n_\phi \cdot i_\phi) \ (\text{mod } \phi_{Omax}) \right] \cdot \Delta\phi_O, \end{aligned}$$

i.e. the position (r_{Oa}, ϕ_a') corresponds to the point (r_{Oa}, ϕ_{Oa}) rotated by the angle ϕ_{di}. Thus, we can precompute the values of the weighting coefficients for the dis-

60

crete angles and use it with special addressing (Lemma 1) during the backprojection (see section 3.1.9).

Definition 12. *The table*

$$WT : [0 : r_{Omax} - 1]_{\mathbb{Z}} \times [0 : \phi_{Omax} - 1]_{\mathbb{Z}} \to \mathbb{R}$$

maps the coordinate of the plane element (r_O, ϕ_O) *to the value of the weighing coefficient for this element*

$$WT[r_O, \phi_O] = \frac{\overline{SO^2}}{\left(\overline{SO} - r_{Oa} \cdot \cos(\phi_{Oa})\right)^2} = \frac{\overline{SO^2}}{\left(\overline{SO} - r_O \cdot \Delta r_O \cdot \cos(\phi_O \cdot \Delta \phi_O)\right)^2}$$

This Weighting Coefficients Table is the same for every plane, thus it is only necessary to calculate the table for one plane. The calculation of the Weighting Coefficients Table is given in Algorithm 5.

Algorithm 5 Calculation of the Weighting Coefficients Table

---

initialize $WT[]$

for $r_O = 0$ to $r_{Omax} - 1$ **do**

  for $\phi_O = 0$ to $\phi_{Omax} - 1$ **do**

    $WT[r_O, \phi_O] \leftarrow \overline{SO^2}/(\overline{SO} - r_{Oa} \cdot \cos(\phi_{Oa}))^2$

  end for

end for

3.1.9 Modified FBP Algorithm

All the definitions, presented in previous sections form now the modified Feldkamp FBP Algorithm called a Cylindrical Algorithm[6] [63]. We formulate the algorithm in the similar form, as the straightforward implementation (Algorithm 1). The Cylindrical Algorithm is described by the Algorithm 6.

At first, the Geometry and the Weighting Coefficients Tables are calculated (Algorithms 5 and 4). Next, for each projection i_ϕ the projection data $P_{d3D}(*, *, i_\phi)$ is filtered row by row and stored in table $FD[*, *, i_\phi]$ (Algorithm 3). The backprojection is performed for each voxel for each projection and consists of the several operations:

---

[6]or Cylindrical FBP Algorithm

1. obtain the address of the voxel for the current projection (z_O, r_O, ϕ) using cyclic rotation (Lemma 1),

2. fetch the coordinates of the intersection p_d and z_d for this voxel from the Geometry Table using the address (z_O, r_O, ϕ_O):

   - p_d is a coordinate in the detector row and can be obtained from the absolute detector address as $INS[z_O, r_O, \phi_O] \pmod{N}$,

   - z_d is a detector row counter and can be computed from the absolute detector address as $\lfloor INS[z_O, r_O, \phi_O]/N \rfloor$,

3. obtain the filtered projection value $FD[p_d, z_d, i_\phi]$,

4. fetch the weighting coefficient $WT[r_O, \phi_O]$ for the current voxel and multiply it with the value $FD[p_d, z_d, i_\phi]$,

5. fetch from the Volume Table $V_c[z_O, r_O, \phi]$, sum this value with the weighted projection value (operation 4) and store it back into the Volume Table.

Thus, during the reconstruction we rotate only the Volume Table, addressing the voxels on a radial element cyclicly using Lemma 1. Other tables, the Geometry and the Weighting Coefficients Tables, are addressed linearly. That is the main advantage of the Cylindrical Algorithm.

The output of the Cylindrical Algorithm is a reconstructed object density. The density values are placed on a cylindrical grid. For the purposes of visualization the interpolation to the Cartesian grid can be carried out.

3.1.10 Analysis of the Cylindrical Algorithm

The analysis of the Cylindrical Algorithm is performed using the following practical considerations:

- the number of elements in one plane is $r_{Omax} \cdot \phi_{Omax} \in O(N^2)$,

- the number of planes is $z_{Omax} \le N$,

Algorithm 6 Cylindrical Algorithm
---
initialize tables $V_c[\,]$, $FD[\,]$, $INS[\,]$ and $WT[\,]$

calculate Weighting Coefficients Table $WT[\,]$ *(Algorithm 5)*

calculate Geometry Table $INS[\,]$ *(Algorithm 4)*

for projection $i_\phi = 0$ to $\phi_{dmax} - 1$ **do**

    Filter detector data and obtain $FD[*,*,i_\phi]$ *(Algorithm 3)*

    for $z_O = 0$ to $z_{Omax} - 1$ **do**

      for $r_O = 0$ to $r_{Omax} - 1$ **do**

        for $\phi_O = 0$ to $\phi_{Omax} - 1$ **do**

                                 (perform the cyclic rotation using Lemma 1)

           $\phi \leftarrow \phi_O - n_\phi \cdot i_\phi \,(\mathrm{mod}\ \phi_{Omax})$

                                   (obtain the horizontal intersection coordinate)

           $p_d \leftarrow INS[z_O,r_O,\phi_O]\,(\mathrm{mod}\ N)$

                                   (obtain the vertical intersection coordinate)

           $z_d \leftarrow \lfloor INS[z_O,r_O,\phi_O]/N \rfloor$

                                   (perform the backprojection)

           $V_c[z_O,r_O,\phi] \leftarrow V_c[z_O,r_O,\phi] + FD[p_d,z_d,i_\phi] \cdot WT[r_O,\phi_O]$

        end for

      end for

    end for

end for

- the number of projections is $\phi_{d\,max} \leq N$,

- the total number of voxels is in $O(N^3)$.

The time complexity of the whole algorithm remains $O(N^4)$ for the reconstruction of the 3D volume from cone-beam projections. The parts of the FBP have the following time complexities:

- the computation of the Geometry Table has time complexity $O(N^3)$;

- the computation of the Weighting Coefficients Table has time complexity $O(N^2)$;

- the filtering using convolution has time complexity $O(N^3)$;

- the backprojection has time complexity $O(N^4)$.

The transformation of the cylindrical volume into the Cartesian coordinates has time complexity $O(N^3)$.

The impact of the cylindrical grid on the image quality in the PC implementation was analyzed by Buck in his thesis [61]. There was reported, that the speed-up due to the introduction of the Cylindrical Algorithm was more than 3 times for $N = 512$ compared to the straightforward implementation of the FBP for 3D CT. For the non-destructive testing [63] this meant a notable reduction of the reconstruction time for industrial tasks, e.g. testing some products for cracks.

The space complexity of the modified algorithm is obtained as follows:

- the Geometry Table $INS[\,]$ has $O(N^3)$ elements,

- the Weighting Coefficients Table $WT[\,]$ has $O(N^2)$ elements,

- the Filtered Projection Table $FD[\,]$ has $\phi_{d\,max} \cdot N^2$ elements (it can be decreased to N^2, storing the filtered data only for the current projection),

- the reconstructed Volume Table $V_c[\,]$ has $O(N^3)$ elements.

Precise values of the required space can be obtained for particular experiment parameter – half-beam opening angle (recall equation for the number of planes (3.1.15)). For the $N = 512$ there are more than $130 \cdot 10^6$ elements in Geometry and Volume tables.

The Geometry, Weighting Coefficients and Volume Tables are accessed sequentially, but the values of Filtered Projection Table are accessed randomly. Thus, the optimization of memory allocation and further modifications of the Cylindrical Algorithm is necessary for the rapid implementation. These changes will be discussed in the next sections during the hardware description.

3.2 Reconstruction Using Parallel Processing

Algorithms improvement and parallel processing technique are the solutions, used to get over the long reconstruction time and big memory requirements.

3.2.1 Overview of the Related Work

Parallel processing systems are based on a number of Processing Elements (PEs). Each PE has its own memory and/or access to the main memory of the system. SIMD[7], MIMD[8] processors and Transputers [68, 69], combined into complex systems, are the examples of the PEs for the CT reconstruction applications in different fields.

Parallel processing uses the distribution of the reconstruction problem between PEs. The partition of reconstruction is based on the four forms of the reconstruction parallelism, defined by Nowinski [70]:

1. *pixel parallelism* (voxel in 3D case) – all pixels are independent of each other,

2. *ray parallelism* – rays can be considered independently during the reconstruction,

---

[7]SIMD: Single-Instruction Stream Multiple-Data Stream
[8]MIMD: Multiple-Instruction Stream Multiple-Data Stream

3. *projection parallelism* – each projection can be handled separately from others, and

4. *operation parallelism* – the low level operations such as additions and multiplications are performed in parallel.

Software Reconstruction Systems

Different CT algorithms implementations were investigated for the large class of the commercially available SIMD and MIMD machines: CM-5, iPSC/2, Intel Paragon, Alpha and Cray [8, 9, 10, 63, 71, 72, 73, 74, 75, 76]. Searching for the efficient interconnection schemes, task distributions and communications between PEs are the main aspects of these studies. Almost all works have practical background, and obtained results were used for the real-world medical and NDT applications. Among the manufactures of the complete CT solutions, that use multiprocessor systems for the 3D reconstruction, are the IZFP Saarbrücken [6, 8, 62, 71], Hapeg [77] and SKYSCAN [7].

Hardware Reconstruction Systems

Several dedicated hardware implementations were proposed for the reconstruction. The PEs can be presented either by Digital Signal Processors (DSPs) or by the custom designs implemented in the Field-Programmable Gate Arrays (FPGAs) or Application-Specific Integrated Circuits (ASICs).

A structure made from the DSPs connected into the hypercube was proposed for the FBP and ART reconstructions [78, 79]. Analyses of the suitable DSPs were made in [16, 80], investigating the characteristics of such processors and their performance applying for the FBP task. As DSPs are optimized for the multiply/accumulate instructions, high performance of such hardware systems was reported. Such systems provided the 2D images reconstruction from the fan-beam projections and constructing the 3D volume from such images.

The custom hardware designs compete with DSPs and general-purpose processors because of the flexibility in control and computation. The earlier examples of

66

the VLSI structures for the CT are given in [14, 15], where the geometry calculations with interpolation and 2D backprojection were implemented in VLSI as a pipelined structure. Optimal realization of the inner products in the FBP algorithm was studied in [13], where different accumulation and multiplication stages were made for the fast 2D reconstruction.

Some studies applied the computer graphics [50] and the specialized volume rendering hardware [81] to solve the reconstruction problems in medical applications. The effective implementation of the iterative reconstruction techniques (ART, SART) was reported.

The pipelined structure on ASIC for the reconstruction of 2D images was build by Agi et. al. [17] and with the multi-DSP system applied for the reconstruction task [18]. Projection filtering using Fast Fourier Transform (FFT) and dataflow management were done by DSPs, whereas the backprojection was made by the pipelined structures on VLSI chips with external memory.

Development of the FPGA technology opened new perspectives for the reconstruction hardware and the new reconfigurable systems were developed [21, 22]. These solutions provide the fast reconstruction for different fields of tomography applications. The great speed-up (compared to the workstation) was achieved in one of the dedicated works for the 2D parallel-beam FBP by using the commercially available board with Xilinx FPGAs [19]. The floating-point calculations were transformed into the fixed-point with theoretical estimation of the error. Filtered backprojection using pre-filtered data was implemented as parallel balanced pipelined architecture with on-chip and external memory.

3.2.2 System Design Considerations

All works perform either fan-beam 2D reconstruction, or combining the 3D volume from the obtained 2D images. None of the currently proposed and developed hardware systems provide the "on-chip" solution (all stages of the algorithm) for the 3D cone-beam FBP reconstruction for the purposes of industrial NDT.

Studies in the field of the hardware reconstruction pointed out, that:

- a modification of the reconstruction algorithm must be performed in order to satisfy the constraints of the applied hardware, e.g. limited bandwidth of the memory system;

- the selected number system for the calculations has impact on the speed of the reconstruction, e.g. fixed-point arithmetic [19] or sign / logarithm number system [13];

- pipelining of the calculations and parallel data streams processing give a fast reconstruction flow.

3.2.3 Hardware Base

Field-Programmable Gate Array (FPGA) is an integrated circuit that can be bought off the shelf and reconfigured by hardware designers themselves. FPGAs offer a lot of advantages for many kinds of applications. The internal structure of the FPGA provides resources for building high performance data processing systems. FPGAs can implement VLSI parts (over 10^6 gate equivalents) within a single device. Among the market FPGA products from Altera, Atmel, Lattice and Xilinx the decision to use of Xilinx FPGAs [82] for system design was made based on the following factors:

- high density and functionality of the current Xilinx FPGA devices;

- large number of available libraries and Intellectual Property (IP) cores: optimized adders, multipliers, dividers etc;

- large number of accompanying programs for the design: Logic Simulator, FPGA Editor, Core Generator, FloorPlanner etc;

- full description of the FPGA devices.

The detailed description of the Xilinx FPGAs can be found in [83]. The manufacturer provides highly optimized implementations of the standard design modules, such as pipelined adders, multipliers, filters, standard interfaces etc.

A tool-independent VHSIC (Very High Speed Integrated Circuit) Hardware Description Language – VHDL [84, 85] is used to describe the structure of a design. Hardware description language allows the specification of the function of designs using programming language forms. The standard libraries, such as IEEE STD_LOGIC and UNISIM, are included and used in the design.

The design is implemented as a "system on-chip" with external SDRAMs and FIFOs. This architecture is validated via gate-level synthesis for Xilinx Virtex II FPGA and emulated on a ModelSIM XE 5.2 simulator [86, 87]. These low-level experiments provided timing and complexity estimates for the proposed design.

3.3 Conclusion

This chapter provided one of the practical reconstruction algorithm for the cone-beam tomography that is currently used in the NDT field [6, 8, 63]. The overview of the fast parallel reconstruction solutions showed the techniques of the fast computations including hardware structures. Some requirements were pointed out for the fast hardware reconstruction, including the hardware base. The description of the reconstruction approach followed by the parallel reconstruction structure will be discussed in the next chapter.

Chapter 4

Formal Description

The previous discussion about the FBP algorithm showed that the main problems in the implementation of the FBP algorithm are the large number of operations, the large memory size and the random access to the Filtered Projection Table.

The modified Algorithm 6 performs the reconstruction using a so-called "projection by projection" reconstruction sequence. In order to minimize the stored amount of data we changed the Cylindrical Algorithm in such a way, that now it performs the reconstruction not "projection by projection", but in "plane by plane" order. With this alternation the reconstruction process requires much less memory. We keep only parts of the Filtered Projection, Volume, Geometry and Weighting Coefficients Tables, that are required to reconstruct the current plane. This reduces the amount of used memory and gives the possibility for an optimization of memory accesses. The side effect of this modification is that the reconstruction now cannot be performed along with the projection measurements.

The following sections of this part present the transformation of the Cylindrical Algorithm. In section 4.1 we start with the sequential backprojection of a radial element in a plane. Then, we introduce the parallelization scheme of the sequential backprojection in section 4.2 and provide the correctness of this scheme. After this, the further modification - pipelining of the parallel backprojection, is presented in section 4.3. Using these modifications we describe the reconstruction of a plane and the reconstruction of a volume in sections 4.4 and 4.5 accordingly.

4.1 Sequential Backprojection

This section presents the description of the sequential reconstruction of a radial element. We consider here only the backprojection process itself. All other calculations, i.e. filtering and geometry computations, will be defined later.

We map the tables of the Cylindrical Algorithm into the corresponding memories. During the description we assume that the required data from these tables are available.

4.1.1 Memories of the Sequential Backprojection

For the sequential backprojection we present the following memories and their correspondence to the tables of the Cylindrical Algorithm. These memories are used here only for the descriptive purposes. The memories of the design are defined later in chapter 5.

The memory EFM is a mapping of the Filtered Projection Table. This memory has capacity of $N^2 \cdot \phi_{dmax}$ elements. For the element (x_d, y_d) $x_d, y_d \in [0 : N-1]_{\mathbb{Z}}$ of the projection $i_\phi \in [0 : \phi_{dmax} - 1]_{\mathbb{Z}}$ the following holds:

$$EFM[N \cdot y_d + x_d, i_\phi] = FD[y_d, x_d, i_\phi].$$

Other memories save the data required for the reconstruction of the particular radial element in a plane. These memories have capacity of ϕ_{Omax} elements. We discuss the reconstruction of the radial element $r_O \in [0 : r_{Omax} - 1]_{\mathbb{Z}}$ in the plane $z_O \in [0 : z_{Omax} - 1]_{\mathbb{Z}}$.

- The weighting memory WTM consists of the elements of the Weighting Coefficients Table

$$WTM[\phi_O] = WT[z_O, r_O, \phi_O] \ \forall \phi_O.$$

- The intersect memory $INSM$ consists of the elements of the Geometry Table

$$INSM[\phi_O] = INS[z_O, r_O, \phi_O] \ \forall \phi_O.$$

- The volume memory VM consist of the elements of the Volume Table

$$VM[\phi_O] = V_c[z_O, r_O, \phi_O] \ \forall \phi_O.$$

4.1.2 Sequential Backprojection Flow

Using the above defined memories we can express the backprojection of a radial element as follows. Assume the reconstruction of the radial element $r_O \in [0 : r_{Omax} - 1]_{\mathbb{Z}}$ in the plane $z_O \in [0 : z_{Omax} - 1]_{\mathbb{Z}}$. Recall the description of the Cylindrical Algorithm in section 3.1.9. We repeat here the backprojection step:

for $i_\phi = 0$ to $\phi_{dmax} - 1$ **do**

$\quad$ ...

$\quad$ **for** $\phi_O = 0$ to $\phi_{Omax} - 1$ **do**

$\qquad p_d \leftarrow INS[z_O, r_O, \phi_O] \,(\text{mod } N)$

$\qquad z_d \leftarrow \lfloor INS[z_O, r_O, \phi_O]/N \rfloor$

$\qquad V_c[z_O, r_O, (\phi_O - n_\phi \cdot i_\phi) \,(\text{mod } \phi_{Omax})] \leftarrow V_c[z_O, r_O,$

$\qquad (\phi_O - n_\phi \cdot i_\phi) \,(\text{mod } \phi_{Omax})] + FD[p_d, z_d, i_\phi] \cdot WT[r_O, \phi_O]$

$\quad$ **end for**

end for

We write this part of the algorithm now in memory notation (from previous section) as

for $i_\phi = 0$ to $\phi_{dmax} - 1$ **do**

$\quad$ **for** $\phi_O = 0$ to $\phi_{Omax} - 1$ **do**

$\qquad VM[(\phi_O - n_\phi \cdot i_\phi) \,(\text{mod } \phi_{Omax})] \leftarrow VM[(\phi_O - n_\phi \cdot i_\phi) \,(\text{mod } \phi_{Omax})]$

$\qquad\qquad\qquad\qquad\qquad + EFM\left[INSM[\phi_O], i_\phi\right] \cdot WTM[\phi_O]$

$\quad$ **end for**

end for

Setting

$$\psi := (\phi_O - n_\phi \cdot i_\phi) \,(\text{mod } \phi_{Omax})$$

and writing $\phi_O = (\psi + n_\phi \cdot i_\phi) \pmod{\phi_{Omax}}$, we obtain

$$VM[\psi] \;\leftarrow\; VM[\psi] + EFM\Big[INSM[(\psi + n_\phi \cdot i_\phi) \pmod{\phi_{Omax}}], i_\phi\Big] \cdot$$
$$WTM[(\psi + n_\phi \cdot i_\phi) \pmod{\phi_{Omax}}].$$

Consider fixed value $i_\phi \in [0 : \phi_{dmax} - 1]_{\mathbb{Z}}$. The memory location $VM[\psi]$ is updated exactly once, namely by $\phi_O = (\psi + n_\phi \cdot i_\phi) \pmod{\phi_{Omax}}$. It is updated by the solution of the equation

$$\psi = (\phi_O - n_\phi \cdot i_\phi) \pmod{\phi_{Omax}}.$$

There can be infinitely many solutions because of the modulo computation

$$(\psi + n_\phi \cdot i_\phi) \pmod{\phi_{Omax}} + k \cdot \phi_{Omax}, \quad k \in \mathbb{Z} \setminus \{0\}.$$

Whereas the loop for ϕ_O is generated for $\phi_O \in [0 : \phi_{Omax} - 1]_{\mathbb{Z}}$ and $n_\phi \in \mathbb{Z}_{\geq 1}$, we have only one solution ψ.

Finally, the update of each location in memory $VM[]$ can be rewritten setting

$$\phi' := (\phi_O + n_\phi \cdot i_\phi) \pmod{\phi_{Omax}}$$

as a sum

$$VM[\phi_O] := \sum_{i_\phi=0}^{\phi_{dmax}-1} EFM\Big[INSM[\phi'], i_\phi\Big] \cdot WTM[\phi']. \qquad (4.1.1)$$

We write now the part of the backprojection of a radial element:

for $\phi_O = 0$ to $\phi_{Omax} - 1$ **do**
$\quad VM[\phi_O] \leftarrow \sum_{i_\phi=0}^{\phi_{dmax}-1} EFM\Big[INSM[\phi'], i_\phi\Big] \cdot WTM[\phi']$
end for

Equation (4.1.1) is a straightforward implementation of the backprojection of a radial element. We address memory VM linearly, whereas other memories are accessed with the counter after cyclic rotation. This will be the model of the backprojection of one voxel on a radial element. Later we will show that the parallel and the pipelined parallel backprojections schemes can be transformed into this model.

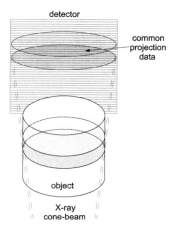

Figure 4.1: Projection of the two planes into the detector.

4.2 Parallel Backprojection

The speed-up of the sequential backprojection is done by re-scheduling of the operations and the correspondent modification of the memory structure. We describe how the sequential backprojection is transformed into the parallel backprojection.

4.2.1 Selection of the Parallelization Method

The reconstruction of several planes in parallel requires the redundancy of the filtered projection data, because the planes can be projected into the same region of the detector (see Figure 4.1). Thus, this common data will be accessed during the reconstruction of each plane. This requires a complex control and scheduling during the reconstruction.

For the same reason the parallel backprojection of several radial elements in one plane can not be performed without the scheduling of the accesses to the common data, required to reconstruct these radial elements.

The parallel reconstruction of the radial element is an effective way to speed-up the reconstruction. During the backprojection all ϕ_{dmax} projections are accessed sequentially and independently from each other. This is used in the parallelization of the backprojection. All projections are divided into several groups. Each group contains an equal number of projections. The accesses inside these groups are performed sequentially, while the accesses to the groups are done in parallel.

Let b be the number of groups of the projections. Each group has

$$p := \frac{\phi_{dmax}}{b}$$

projections, where ϕ_{dmax} and b are selected in such a way, that p is a power of two. The index $i \in [0 : b-1]_{\mathbb{Z}}$ will denote now the number of the group and the index $j \in [0 : p-1]_{\mathbb{Z}}$ will be used inside this group. Obviously, for some projection j in the group i we can obtain the value i_ϕ as follows

$$i_\phi := i \cdot p + j.$$

Each group of projections is stored in a separate memory, thus we have b such memories. These memories are required to reorder the weighted values from b projections, because they correspond to the different voxels. These memories are accessed in parallel using a common address. This address is taken from the intersect memory. The intersect memory is accessed sequentially with $\phi_O \in [0 : \phi_{Omax} - 1]_{\mathbb{Z}}$. With each access to the filtered projections we fetch b filtered values simultaneously. These values are weighted with a common weighting coefficient and stored in intermediate memories. After $\phi_{Omax} \cdot b$ many values were fetched and weighted, they are accumulated. This process is repeated for p times.

There is a possibility to avoid the additional intermediate memories by using b copies of the intersect and weighting memories. The access address for the intersect and weighting memories must be precomputed for each voxel. But the side effect of this structure is, that if we will use the dynamic memory for the filtered data, the output values will be non-synchronous. So, using the common address for all external memories we have the identical memory functioning, i.e. all accesses and memory control are identical for all chips.

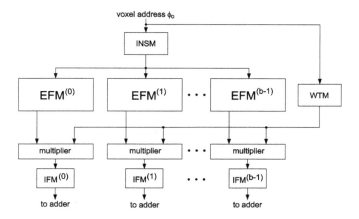

Figure 4.2: Memory structure of the parallel backprojection.

4.2.2 Memories of the Parallel Backprojection

The schematic of the memory structure for the parallel backprojection is depicted on Figure 4.2. The memories $INSM$, WTM and VM stay the same as for the sequential backprojection. By $VM^{\{j\}}$ we will denote the contents of the memory VM after the round j. This is used for the description of the accumulation.

We introduce a new notation for the memories, that store the filtered projection data. There are now b such memories. By $EFM^{(i)}$ we denote the memory, that consists of the projections of the ith group. Each projection has N^2 elements. The $EFM^{(i)}$ corresponds to the EFM in the following way

$$EFM^{(i)}[*, j] \Longleftrightarrow EFM[*, i \cdot p + j] \quad j \in [0 : p-1]_{\mathbb{Z}} \quad i \in [0 : b-1]_{\mathbb{Z}}. \quad (4.2.1)$$

Obviously, the total capacity of all b memories $EFM^{(i)}$ is equal to the capacity of the EFM memory from the sequential model.

We introduce a new memory structure, that is required for the parallel implementation of the backprojection. Before the summation, the weighted input data is reordered using the group index i and the projection index j. The data from the $EFM^{(i)}$ is stored in the ith intermediate filtered memory denoted by the $IFM^{(i)}$. Each of these memories stores ϕ_{Omax} elements.

77

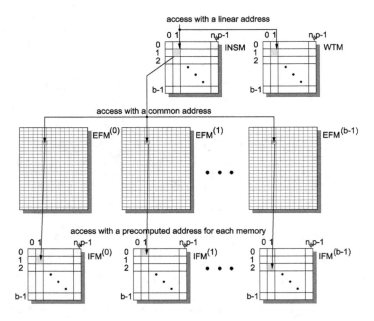

Figure 4.3: Access to the different memories of the parallel backprojection. Recall that $\phi_{Omax} = n_\phi \cdot \phi_{dmax} = n_\phi \cdot p \cdot b$. The example on this figure uses values $\phi_O = n_\phi \cdot p + 1$ and $j = 0$.

4.2.3 Parallel Backprojection Flow

Consider the reconstruction of the radial element $r_O \in [0 : r_{Omax} - 1]_\mathbb{Z}$ in the plane $z_O \in [0 : z_{Omax} - 1]_\mathbb{Z}$. The backprojection of the whole radial element is divided into p rounds with the round counter j. Each round consists of two stages: processing of the filtered data and accumulation.

Processing of the Filtered Data

The memory *INSM* is accessed sequentially using ϕ_O as an address (see Figure 4.3). This is done for all ϕ_{Omax} elements in one round j. The values of the intersect memory are used as the common addresses for all $EFM^{(i)}$ memories:

$$EFM^{(i)}[INSM[\phi_O], j] \quad \forall i.$$

The filtered projection data, fetched from the memories $EFM^{(i)}$, are multiplied with the weighting coefficients. These coefficients are fetched from the memory WTM using the address ϕ_O. The memory WTM is accessed sequentially as the memory $INSM$. The products of the multiplication are stored in the intermediate filtered memories $IFM^{(i)}$

$$IFM^{(i)}[\phi'] := EFM^{(i)}\left[INSM[\phi_O], j\right] \cdot WTM[\phi_O] \quad \forall i \qquad (4.2.2)$$

using the address

$$\phi' := (\phi_O - n_\phi \cdot (i \cdot p + j)) \pmod{\phi_{Omax}}.$$

This is called a *reordering process* – sequentially accessed filtered data from the b memories are stored in the corresponding intermediate memories. The address in these memories depends on the current round j and the index of the projection group i. The following Lemma provides the correctness of the data reordering.

Lemma 2. *Let* $\phi := (\phi_O + n_\phi \cdot (i \cdot p + j)) \pmod{\phi_{Omax}}$ *for* $\phi_O \in [0 : \phi_{Omax} - 1]_{\mathbb{Z}}$. *For an arbitrary round* $j \in [0 : p - 1]_{\mathbb{Z}}$ *the following holds*

$$IFM^{(i)}[\phi_O] = EFM^{(i)}\left[INSM[\phi], j\right] \cdot WTM[\phi] \quad \forall i. \qquad (4.2.3)$$

The Equation (4.2.3) describes the parallel access to the b memories $EFM^{(i)}$. Each access to i^{th} memory is performed as for the sequential backprojection (4.1.1). We compute ϕ for the round j. Then we access all memories $EFM^{(i)}$ and write the fetched values into the corresponding intermediate memories $IFM^{(i)}$. The write address for these memories is ϕ_O.

Proof. We express the index ϕ_O using the index ϕ as

$$\phi_O = (\phi - n_\phi \cdot (i \cdot p + j)) \pmod{\phi_{Omax}}.$$

Inserting ϕ_O into the the Equation (4.2.3) gives the Equation (4.2.2)

$$IFM^{(i)}[(\phi - n_\phi \cdot (i \cdot p + j)) \pmod{\phi_{Omax}}] = EFM^{(i)}\left[INSM[\phi], j\right] \cdot WTM[\phi]. \quad \square$$

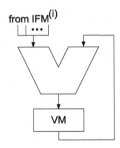

from IFM$^{(i)}$

VM

Figure 4.4: Accumulation stage for parallel backprojection.

After the round j the intermediate memories consist of the weighted filtered elements from b projections. These elements are used during the accumulation stage of the parallel backprojection.

Accumulation

During the accumulation stage all b memories $IFM^{(i)}$ are accessed in parallel with the common address $\phi_O \in [0 : \phi_{O_{max}} - 1]_{\mathbb{Z}}$. The data, fetched from the intermediate memories are accumulated with the result of the previous round (Figure 4.4). The result is stored in the volume memory VM

$$VM^{\{j\}}[\phi_O] := \sum_{i=0}^{b-1} IFM^{(i)}[\phi_O] + VM^{\{j-1\}}[\phi_O]. \tag{4.2.4}$$

We ensure that before the first accumulation ($j = 0$) all elements of the memory VM are equal to zero. Equation (4.2.4) means that in the round j we accumulate the weighted filtered data from the projections ($i \cdot p + j$) for all i. After p rounds the memory VM will store the result of the backprojection of a radial element.

4.2.4 Correctness of the Parallel Backprojection

The correctness of the parallel backprojection of a radial element is given by the following Theorem.

Theorem 2. *The result of the parallel backprojection of a radial element in a plane is the same as the result of the sequential backprojection of this radial element.*

80

Proof. We will show that the parallel backprojection, described by Equations (4.2.3) and (4.2.4) can be transformed into the sequential backprojection. We discuss the reconstruction of the radial element $r_O \in [0 : r_{Omax} - 1]_{\mathbb{Z}}$ in the plane $z_O \in [0 : z_{Omax} - 1]_{\mathbb{Z}}$.

Let $\phi := (\phi_O + n_\phi \cdot (i \cdot p + j)) \,(\mathrm{mod}\ \phi_{Omax})$. Applying Lemma 2 to the sum

$$\sum_{i=0}^{b-1} IFM^{(i)}[\phi_O]$$

from the Equation (4.2.4), for all p rounds we obtain the following:

$$VM^{\{p\}}[\phi_O] = \sum_{j=0}^{p-1}\sum_{i=0}^{b-1} EFM^{(i)}\Big[INSM[\phi], j\Big] \cdot WTM[\phi].$$

Using the correspondence (4.2.1) of the $EFM^{(i)}$ to the memory EFM we write

$$VM^{\{p\}}[\phi_O] = \sum_{j=0}^{p-1}\sum_{i=0}^{b-1} EFM\Big[INSM[\phi], i \cdot p + j\Big] \cdot WTM[\phi].$$

The double sum is nothing else than the sum of the weighted data over all projections. Recall that $i_\phi := i \cdot p + j$. Introducing the new variable

$$\phi' = (\phi_O + n_\phi \cdot i_\phi) \,(\mathrm{mod}\ \phi_{Omax})$$

and combining two sums we have (see (4.1.1))

$$VM^{\{p\}}[\phi_O] = \sum_{i_\phi=0}^{\phi_{dmax}-1} EFM\Big[INSM[\phi'], i_\phi\Big] \cdot WTM[\phi']. \quad \square$$

4.3   Pipelined Parallel Backprojection

The parallelization scheme described in the previous section speeds up the backprojection in the Cylindrical Algorithm. This modification can be optimized using the pipelining technique. During the parallel backprojection, when the fetch of the filtered data is performed, the part of the resources for the accumulation stage is idle. This situation is changed when we try to re-schedule the backprojection using pipelining.

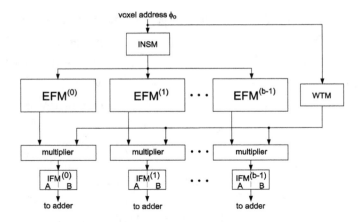

Figure 4.5: Memory structure of the pipelined parallel backprojection of a radial element.

4.3.1 Memories of the Pipelined Backprojection

The memory structure of the parallel backprojection must be changed in order to perform the pipelined computations. The memory structure of the pipelined parallel backprojection is depicted on Figure 4.5.

For the pipelining we use the doubled memory structure. It consists of two memories with equal capacity. These memories are denoted for simplicity by A and B. For the pipelining process these memories are used in the following way: one memory is available for reading, another - for writing, and then the functions of these memories are interchanged.

The intermediate filtered memory uses this doubled structure – there are totaly $2 \cdot b$ such memories. By $IFM_{Cr}^{(i,j)}$ we denote the memory for reading access and by $IFM_{Cw}^{(i,j)}$ – for writing access. The type of the access to the internal memories is defined by the index j

$$IFM_{Cr}^{(i,j)} = \begin{cases} IFM_A^{(i)} & j \text{ is odd} \\ IFM_B^{(i)} & j \text{ is even} \end{cases}, \quad IFM_{Cw}^{(i,j)} = \begin{cases} IFM_A^{(i)} & j \text{ is even} \\ IFM_B^{(i)} & j \text{ is odd} \end{cases}.$$

Such construction of memories provides the following property

$$IFM_{Cr}^{(i,j+1)}[\phi_O] := IFM_{Cw}^{(i,j)}[\phi_O] \quad \forall \phi_O. \tag{4.3.1}$$

82

In another words, the data that was written in the round j is available for reading in the round $(j+1)$.

There are two memories that are used to store the intermediate result of the back-projection and one memory is used to store the final result of the backprojection. The memories, used for the intermediate computations are denoted by $VM_{Cr}^{(s)}$ and $VM_{Cw}^{(s)}$. They are used for reading and writing accesses, accordingly.

$$VM_{Cr}^{(s)} = \begin{cases} VM_A & s \text{ is odd} \\ VM_B & s \text{ is even} \end{cases} \qquad VM_{Cw}^{(s)} = \begin{cases} VM_A & s \text{ is even} \\ VM_B & s \text{ is odd} \end{cases}$$

The memory that stores the final result of the reconstruction is denoted by VM_O.

Other memories are the same as defined in section 4.2.2. The memory $EFM^{(i)}$ is used for the filtered data, the $INSM$ for geometry data and the WTM for the weighting coefficients.

4.3.2 Pipelined Parallel Reconstruction Flow

We describe the pipelined parallel backprojection of a radial element. The pipelined schedule of the backprojection of several radial elements will be presented later.

Consider the reconstruction of the radial element $r_O \in [0 : r_{Omax} - 1]_{\mathbb{Z}}$ in the plane $z_O \in [0 : z_{Omax} - 1]_{\mathbb{Z}}$. The backprojection of the radial element is performed in p rounds. In each round j the filtered data is fetched from the b memories $EFM^{(i)}$ using the values from the intersect memory as the addresses:

$$EFM^{(i)}\left[INSM[\phi_O], j\right] \quad \forall i, \forall \phi_O.$$

The weighting memory is also accessed sequentially with ϕ_O in each round j. The filtered data from each memory $EFM^{(i)}$ is multiplied with the weighting coefficient $WTM[\phi_O]$. Using the address

$$\phi' := (\phi_O - n_\phi \cdot (i \cdot p + j)) \pmod{\phi_{Omax}}$$

the ith product value is stored in the ith intermediate memory $IFM_{Cw}^{(i,j)}$ as

$$IFM_{Cw}^{(i,j)}[\phi'] := EFM^{(i)}\left[INSM[\phi_O], j\right] \cdot WTM[\phi_O] \quad \forall i. \tag{4.3.2}$$

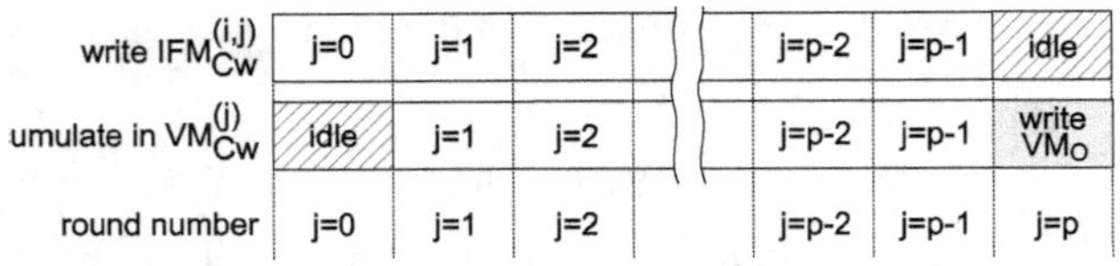

write IFM$_{Cw}^{(i,j)}$	j=0	j=1	j=2		j=p-2	j=p-1	idle
umulate in VM$_{Cw}^{(j)}$	idle	j=1	j=2		j=p-2	j=p-1	write VM$_O$
round number	j=0	j=1	j=2		j=p-2	j=p-1	j=p

Figure 4.6: Pipelined parallel backprojection of a radial element.

This is done for all b memories $IFM_{Cw}^{(i,j)}$ in parallel for p rounds. Lemma 2 provides the correctness of the data reordering.

Data, that is fetched and reordered in the round j, is accumulated in the round $(j+1)$. Figure 4.6 provides the graphical description of the pipelining process. For the description we use the following property of the doubled memory structure

$$VM_{Cr}^{(j+1)}[\phi_O] := VM_{Cw}^{(j)}[\phi_O]. \tag{4.3.3}$$

In each round $j \in [1 : p-1]_{\mathbb{Z}}$ the data from the $IFM_{Cr}^{(i,j)}[\phi_O]$ is accumulated with the previous result, which is found in the memory $VM_{Cr}^{(j)}[\phi_O]$. This sum is stored in the memory $VM_{Cw}^{(j)}$. This is done for each $\phi_O \in [0 : \phi_{Omax} - 1]_{\mathbb{Z}}$

$$VM_{Cw}^{(j)}[\phi_O] := \sum_{i=0}^{b-1} IFM_{Cr}^{(i,j)}[\phi_O] + VM_{Cr}^{(j)}[\phi_O]. \tag{4.3.4}$$

In the first round of accumulation all elements in the memory $VM_{Cr}^{(1)}[\phi_O]$ must be equal to zero. Using the property (4.3.3) this is expressed as

$$VM_{Cw}^{(0)}[\phi_O] := 0 \quad \forall \phi_O. \tag{4.3.5}$$

After p backprojection rounds all required data are fetched from the filtered projection memory. To obtain the result of the backprojection one more round is needed, because weighted and reordered data from the round $j = p - 1$ was not yet accumulated. During this additional round, the result of the backprojection is stored in the memory VM_O (Figure 4.7)

$$VM_O[\phi_O] := \sum_{i=0}^{b-1} IFM_{Cr}^{(i,p)}[\phi_O] + VM_{Cr}^{(p)}[\phi_O]. \tag{4.3.6}$$

84

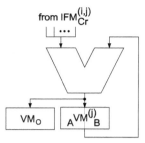

from IFM$_{Cr}^{(i,j)}$

VM$_O$

A VM$^{(i)}$ B

Figure 4.7: Accumulation stage for the pipelined parallel backprojection of a radial element.

The data fetch and the accumulation are carried out in p rounds, but accumulation starts later, in the round $j = 1$. Counting the additional round, we have totaly $(p+1)$ rounds for the backprojection of a radial element. Later, when the whole plane will be reconstructed using the pipelined parallel backprojection scheme, we will show that each radial element is reconstructed in p rounds. This is possible, because the idle rounds at the beginning of the backprojection of the radial elements are removed.

4.3.3 Correctness of the Pipelined Parallel Backprojection

The correctness of the presented pipelined parallel reconstruction, described by the Equations (4.3.2)-(4.3.6), is provided by the following Theorem.

Theorem 3. *The result of the pipelined parallel backprojection of a radial element is the same as the result of the sequential backprojection of the same radial element.*

Proof. We will show that the Equations (4.3.2) - (4.3.6) can be transformed into the non-pipelined parallel backprojection of a radial element (from section 4.2).

The contents of the memory $VM_{Cr}^{(p)}$ is the sum of the weighted filtered data fetched in the $(p-1)$ rounds. Using that the memory elements of the $VM_{Cr}^{(1)}$ are equal to zero (4.3.5), the contents of the memory $VM_{Cr}^{(p)}$ is expressed as

$$VM_{Cr}^{(p)}[\phi_O] = VM_{Cw}^{(p-1)}[\phi_O] = \sum_{j=1}^{p-1}\sum_{i=0}^{b-1} IFM_{Cr}^{(i,j)}[\phi_O].$$

85

We plug this into the Equation (4.3.6) and obtain the following formula

$$
\begin{aligned}
VM_O[\phi_O] &= \sum_{i=0}^{b-1} IFM_{Cr}^{(i,p)}[\phi_O] + VM_{Cr}^{(p)}[\phi_O] \\
&= \sum_{i=0}^{b-1} IFM_{Cr}^{(i,p)}[\phi_O] + \sum_{j=1}^{p-1}\sum_{i=0}^{b-1} IFM_{Cr}^{(i,j)}[\phi_O] \\
&= \sum_{j=1}^{p}\sum_{i=0}^{b-1} IFM_{Cr}^{(i,j)}[\phi_O].
\end{aligned}
$$

The last equation can be represented using the property (4.3.1) as

$$
\begin{aligned}
VM_O[\phi_O] &= \sum_{j=1}^{p}\sum_{i=0}^{b-1} IFM_{Cw}^{(i,j-1)}[\phi_O] \\
&= \sum_{j=0}^{p-1}\sum_{i=0}^{b-1} IFM_{Cw}^{(i,j)}[\phi_O].
\end{aligned}
$$

Applying Lemma 2 to the new notation $(IFM_{Cw}^{(i,j)})$ we express now the data, stored in the memory $IFM_{Cw}^{(i,j)}$ as

$$
IFM_{Cw}^{(i,j)}[\phi_O] = EFM^{(i)}\Big[INSM[\phi], j\Big] \cdot WTM[\phi]
$$

where the index ϕ is expressed as $\phi := (\phi_O - n_\phi \cdot (i \cdot p + j)) \,(\mathrm{mod}\ \phi_{Omax})$. These data are accumulated in the memory VM_O as follows:

$$
VM_O[\phi_O] = \sum_{j=0}^{p-1}\sum_{i=0}^{b-1} EFM^{(i)}\Big[INSM[\phi], j\Big] \cdot WTM[\phi].
$$

The obtained equation is a parallel backprojection of a radial element, described in section 4.2.3. By Theorem 2 the result of the parallel backprojection of a radial element is equal to the result of the sequential backprojection of the same radial element. □

4.4 Pipelined Reconstruction of a Plane

Using the pipelined parallel backprojection of a radial element we describe now the reconstruction of a plane.

The reconstruction of a plane consists of the backprojection of the radial elements and the geometry computations. The geometry data, required for the reconstruction of the radial element is computed before the backprojection of this element.

4.4.1 Geometry Computations

The significant part of the reconstruction are the geometry computations. The Cylindrical Algorithm increases the efficiency storing the pre-computed geometry information, the intersect addresses and the weighting coefficients, in the Geometry and Weighting tables accordingly. But this large amount of memory ($O(N^3)$) is not efficient for the hardware reconstruction.

In our design we use the Geometry and Weighting tables only partially. We compute and store only those elements of tables, that are required to reconstruct the voxels of one radial element. This modification of the Cylindrical Algorithm significantly decreases the amount of memory required for the geometry data. The reconstruction schedule allows to perform the geometry computations in parallel with the backprojection of the radial element.

The geometry and weighting tables are stored in the corresponding memories, used during the backprojection (recall their definitions from section 4.1.1). For the reconstruction of a plane we modify these memories. Now, the memories have a doubled structure similar to those described in section 4.3.1.

The Intersect memory consists of two memories, A and B. Each memory inside this structure has a capacity of ϕ_{Omax} elements. By $INSM_{Cr}^{(s)}$ we denote the Intersect memory that is accessed for reading and by $INSM_{Cw}^{(s)}$ – for writing. The internal memories are selected depending on the parameter s

$$INSM_{Cr}^{(s)} = \begin{cases} INSM_A & s \text{ is odd} \\ INSM_B & s \text{ is even} \end{cases} \quad \text{and } INSM_{Cw}^{(s)} = \begin{cases} INSM_A & s \text{ is even} \\ INSM_B & s \text{ is odd} \end{cases}.$$

The Weighting memory has the similar structure as the Intersect memory. By $WTM_{Cr}^{(s)}$ and $WTM_{Cw}^{(s)}$ we denote memories for reading and writing accesses accordingly:

$$WTM_{Cr}^{(s)} = \begin{cases} WTM_A & \text{s is odd} \\ WTM_B & \text{s is even} \end{cases}, \quad WTM_{Cw}^{(s)} = \begin{cases} WTM_A & \text{s is even} \\ WTM_B & \text{s is odd} \end{cases}.$$

The above defined memories have the following property

$$INSM_{Cr}^{(s+1)}[\phi_O] := INSM_{Cw}^{(s)}[\phi_O]$$

and

$$WTM_{Cr}^{(s+1)}[\phi_O] := WTM_{Cw}^{(s)}[\phi_O] \quad \forall \phi_O.$$

The computation of the geometry data – intersect coordinates and weighting coefficients will be described in section 5.6, where the construction of the whole Geometry Computations Unit will be discussed.

4.4.2 Reconstruction Schedule

For the description of the reconstruction schedule we use the notation presented in section 4.3.

Consider the reconstruction of the plane $z_O \in [0 : z_{Omax} - 1]_{\mathbb{Z}}$. Each radial element is reconstructed using the pipelined parallel backprojection. For the reconstruction of several radial elements the backprojection flow (section 4.3) is modified in the following way.

The reconstruction flow is presented in Algorithm 7. In the loop for all radial elements (lines 2-18) two processes are performed in parallel: geometry computations (lines 3-5) and the backprojection of the radial element (lines 6-17). The graphical representation of this flow is depicted on Figure 4.8(a).

Before the reconstruction of a plane starts, the geometry data (intersect points and weighting coefficients) are computed (line 1). These data are used in the reconstruction of the first radial element ($r_O = 0$). During the geometry computations the geometry data for the next radial element are written into two memories: intersect memory $INSM_{Cw}^{(r_O)}$ and weighting memory $WTM_{Cw}^{(r_O)}$. Selection of the internal memories is done using the index r_O of the current radial element.

Algorithm 7 Reconstruction of a Plane

Require: memories $EFM^{(i)}$ consist of filtered projection data

1: compute geometry data for $r_O = 0$

2: **for** $r_O = 0$ to $r_{O max} - 1$ **do**

3:     **if** $r_O < r_{O max} - 1$ **then**

4:         compute geometry data for $r_O + 1$

5:     **end if**

6:     **for** $j = 0$ to $p - 1$ in parallel for each group of projections i **do**

7:         **for** $\phi_O = 0$ to $\phi_{O max} - 1$ **do**

8:             $\phi \leftarrow (\phi_O - n_\phi \cdot (i \cdot p + j)) \,(\mathrm{mod}\ \phi_{O max})$

9:             $IFM_{Cw}^{(i,j)}[\phi] \leftarrow EFM^{(i)}\left[INSM_{Cr}^{(r_O)}[\phi_O], j\right] \cdot WTM_{Cr}^{(r_O)}[\phi_O]$

10:           **if** $j = 0$ **then**

11:              $VM_{Cw}^{(j)}[\phi_O] \leftarrow 0$

12:              $VM_O[\phi_O] \leftarrow \sum_{i=0}^{b-1} IFM_{Cr}^{(i,j)}[\phi_O] + VM_{Cr}^{(j)}[\phi_O]$

13:           **else**

14:              $VM_{Cw}^{(j)}[\phi_O] \leftarrow \sum_{i=0}^{b-1} IFM_{Cr}^{(i,j)}[\phi_O] + VM_{Cr}^{(j)}[\phi_O]$

15:           **end if**

16:         **end for**

17:     **end for**

18: **end for**

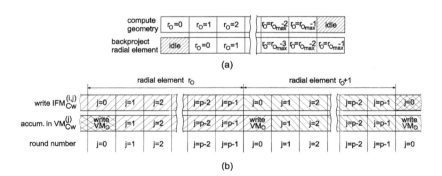

Figure 4.8: Reconstruction of a plane. (a) Two processes of the reconstruction - geometry computation and backprojection. (b) Backprojection of several radial elements.

The reconstruction of a radial element is performed as it was described in section 4.3. The only change for the pipelined parallel reconstruction of a plane is made in the schedule in order to eliminate the idle rounds:

the reconstruction of the new radial element starts with the last round of the backprojection of the previous radial element.

This last round is denoted by "write VM_O" on Figure 4.8(b). During this round the memory $VM_{Cw}^{(0)}$ is cleared. This is done in order to add zeros in the next round, when the accumulation for the new radial element starts (line 14). Thus, the requirement for the pipelined parallel backprojection of a radial element is fulfilled (section 4.3.2).

At this point, we discuss the geometry computations on the abstract level, without any specification. They will be formally defined in section 5.6. Now, we assume that the geometry computations for one radial element are performed not faster than the backprojection of a radial element.

4.5 Reconstruction of the Volume

To describe the pipelined parallel reconstruction of the whole volume we will use the previously introduced reconstruction of a radial element and a plane. We have described all processes and requirements for the reconstruction of a plane, except how the data is filtered and stored in memories $EFM^{(i)}$.

We will analyze the consumption of the projection memory of the Cylindrical Algorithm, and introduce memory structure for the filtered projection data. At the end of this section we will describe the pipelined parallel reconstruction of the volume from the cone-beam projections.

4.5.1 Projection of a Plane

The part of the object, that is reconstructed later as a plane, is projected into the region of the detector. The height of this region is a number of detector rows. We will use this information to define the capacity of the filtered projection memory in our design.

Definition 13. *A set of detector rows, that contains the projection of a plane z_O, is defined as*

$$lines(z_O) = \{y_d \mid P_{d3D}[*, y_d, *] \text{ required to reconstruct the plane}$$
$$z_O \in [0 : z_{Omax} - 1]_\mathbb{Z}\}.$$

The cardinality of the set $lines(z_O)$ is a number of detector rows, required for the reconstruction of the plane z_O.

The reconstruction process is started from the upper plane and we move down, reconstructing plane by plane sequentially[1]. For the reconstruction of some plane z_O we need to know how many detector rows were already filtered and used in the reconstruction of the previous planes, that are situated upper than our current plane (see Figure 4.9). Thus, the detector rows which were used to reconstruct planes before the current plane z_O, are defined as

$$Lines(z_O) = \bigcup_{0 \leq z < z_O} lines(z).$$

Definition 14. *A set of detector rows for the reconstruction of the plane z_O, that must be filtered and added to the already available rows is*

$$\Delta lines(z_O) = lines(z_O) \setminus Lines(z_O).$$

The number of detector rows, required for the reconstruction of the plane is dependent on the parameters of the experiment. This will be analyzed later in the evaluation chapter.

---

[1]The reconstruction can be started from the arbitrary plane in the volume and move further in the arbitrary direction (up or down). In this case the table *DLC* must be changed.

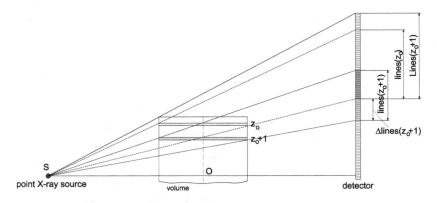

Figure 4.9: Projection of two planes into the detector.

Definition 15. *By* $DLC[z_O]$ *we denote the table*

$$DLC : [0 : z_{Omax} - 1]_{\mathbb{Z}} \rightarrow \mathbb{Z}$$

that maps the coordinate of the plane $z_O \in [0 : z_{Omax} - 1]_{\mathbb{Z}}$ *in the volume to the corresponding value*

$$DLC[z_O] = \begin{cases} \#lines(0) & \text{if } z_O = 0 \\ \#\Delta lines(z_O) & \text{if } z_O \neq 0 \end{cases}$$

computed for some particular half-beam opening angle α.

The first element of this table contains the number of detector rows, that must be filtered initially to start the reconstruction of the volume. We assume[2] that the set $lines(0)$ contains detector rows from $y_d = 0$. The table DLC is mapped into the memory $DLCM$ that contains z_{Omax} elements of the table DLC.

One particular important property of table DLC is that for the real experiment parameters (see chapter 6) the following holds: $DLC[z_O] = 1$ for *almost* all $z_O \geq 1$. There are non-one values, e.g. "zeros" and "twos", but they arise seldom only due to the rounding during the computations. Therefore, in some of the future timing diagrams we only show one case $DLC[z_O] = 1$ for $z_O \geq 1$ for simplicity.

---

[2]In practice we eliminate the unused detector rows and start counting from the first detector row, that contains the projection information.

The maximal number of detector rows, required to reconstruct a plane in the current volume is

$$L_{max} := \max_{z_O \in [0:z_{Omax}-1]_{\mathbb{Z}}} (\#lines(z_O)).$$

Let

$$n_r := 2^{\lceil \log_2(L_{max}) \rceil} \tag{4.5.1}$$

be the number of detector rows, that are stored in the memory. By definition $n_r \geq L_{max}$. Hence, for the reconstruction of each plane the memory will consist of the sufficient amount of filtered detector rows. In chapter 6 we will analyze the impact of the experiment parameters on the value L_{max}.

4.5.2 Filtered Projection Memory

For the minimization of the amount of memory used for the reconstruction, we store only the part of the filtered detector data, which is required for the reconstruction of one plane.

Consider the reconstruction of the plane $z_O \in [0:z_{Omax}-1]_{\mathbb{Z}}$. The filtered detector rows required for the reconstruction of the current plane are stored in the memory structure $EFM^{(i)}$. There are b memories, each consists of n_r filtered detector rows for p projections. The capacity of each ith memory is $n_r \cdot p \cdot N$ elements. The total number of the filtered detector elements available in the system is $n_r \cdot \phi_{dmax} \cdot N$.

For the reconstruction of the next plane $z_O + 1$, the memories $EFM^{(i)}$ are updated. We filter and store $\#\Delta lines(z_O + 1)$ detector rows in the $EFM^{(i)}$. This process is performed in the following way. During the reconstruction the memories $EFM^{(i)}$ are used in each cycle of the backprojection. That's why the input filtered data are stored in the intermediate memories denoted by $EIFM^{(i)}$. Each filtered projection memory $EFM^{(i)}$ has the corresponding intermediate memory $EIFM^{(i)}$. All $EIFM^{(i)}$ together hold data for one detector row $y_d \in [0:N-1]_{\mathbb{Z}}$ for all projections $i_\phi \in [0:\phi_{dmax}-1]_{\mathbb{Z}}$, i.e.

$$EIFM^{(i)}[j \cdot N + x_d] = FD[x_d, y_d, i_\phi] \quad \forall x_d.$$

93

When the detector row is completely filtered (for all projections) and the filtered data is written into the intermediate memories, we wait until the end of the reconstruction of a plane. After this, the data is transferred from the $EIFM^{(i)}$ into the $EFM^{(i)}$ in parallel for all b memories. Using the address of the row $y_d \pmod{n_r}$ the new data is written over the old data that was already stored in memories $EFM^{(i)}$

$$EFM^{(i)}[y_d \pmod{n_r} + x_d, j] \leftarrow EIFM^{(i)}[j \cdot N + x_d] \quad \forall j, y_d, x_d.$$

During the reconstruction of the whole volume with z_{Omax} planes the filtering and data transfer between memories are done for all detector rows $y_d \in [0 : N-1]_{\mathbb{Z}}$.

The correctness of the memory update for the reconstruction of each plane z_O is provided by Lemma 3 in the next section.

4.5.3 Filtering of the Projection Data

The filtering of the projection data is performed using the direct implementation of the convolution. Recall definition of variables from section 2.8. The filtering is a computation of the Filtered Projection Table (3.1.4):

$$FD[x_d, y_d, i_\phi] = d \sum_{k=0}^{N-1} P_{d3D}(k, y_d, i_\phi) h(x_d \cdot d - k \cdot d) \frac{\overline{SO}}{\sqrt{\overline{SO}^2 + p_x^2 + z_y^2}} \quad \forall x_d, y_d, i_\phi$$

which is mapped into the memories $EFM^{(i)}$. The input projection data P_{d3D} must be already pre-weighted

$$P_{d3Dw}(x_d, y_d, i_\phi) = P_{d3D}(x_d, y_d, i_\phi) \cdot \frac{d \cdot \overline{SO}}{\sqrt{\overline{SO}^2 + p_x^2 + z_y^2}}, \quad \forall x_d, y_d, i_\phi.$$

This is included in the preprocessing conditions (section 5.2.2).

Filtering is done for each detector row sequentially for all projections. Each row y_d is filtered and saved into the intermediate memories $EIFM^{(i)}$ (Algorithm 8). After the row is filtered, data from the memories $EIFM^{(i)}$ is transferred into the $EFM^{(i)}$ (Algorithm 9).

Recall the description of the set $lines(z_O)$. For the reconstruction of each plane the corresponding number $\#lines(z_O)$ of filtered detector rows must be available. We

Algorithm 8 Filtering of a Detector Row y_d

1: **for** $i_\phi = 0$ to $\phi_{dmax} - 1$ **do**   *(counter of projections)*

2:     **for** $x_d = 0$ to $N - 1$ **do**   *(counter in a row)*

3:         $i \leftarrow \lfloor i_\phi / p \rfloor$ *(compute the projection's group number)*

4:         $j \leftarrow i_\phi \pmod p$ *(compute the offset in a group)*

5:         $EIFM^{(i)}[j \cdot N + x_d] \leftarrow \sum_{k=0}^{N-1} P_{d3Dw}(k, y_d, i_\phi) h(x_d \cdot d - k \cdot d)$

6:     **end for**

7: **end for**

Algorithm 9 Data Transfer to the Memories $EFM^{(i)}$

1: **for** $j = 0$ to $p - 1$ **do**   *(counter in groups of projections)*

2:     **for** $x_d = 0$ to $N - 1$ **do**   *(counter in a row)*

3:         $EFM^{(i)}[y_d \pmod{n_r} + x_d, j] \leftarrow EIFM^{(i)}[j \cdot N + x_d]$

4:     **end for**

5: **end for**

---

need to add detector rows, that are contained in the set $\Delta lines(z_O)$, to the already filtered rows. Thus, the preparing of the detector rows for the reconstruction of the plane z_O will be the following:

1: **for all** $y_d \in \Delta lines(z_O)$ **do**

2:     filter detector row y_d *(Algorithm 8)*

3:     transfer filtered row into the $EFM^{(i)}$ *(Algorithm 9)*

4: **end for**

The following lemma summarizes the above presented description.

Lemma 3. *The filtered projection data required for the reconstruction of the arbitrary plane z_O is obtained after filtering and adding $\#\Delta lines(z_O)$ detector rows into the memory structure $EFM^{(i)}$.*

Proof. We will prove this Lemma by induction over the planes.

1. Consider the upper plane of the volume ($z_O = 0$). Before the reconstruction of this plane we need to filter and store $\#lines(0)$ detector rows (the value $DLCM[0]$). These processes are described in the Algorithms 8 and 9. By definition

$$\#lines(0) \leq L_{max} \leq n_r.$$

As the memory structure $EFM^{(i)}$ has the total capacity of $n_r \cdot \phi_{d\,max} \cdot N$ elements, the amount of filtered data is not greater than this capacity. Thus, all projection data, required for the reconstruction of the upper plane will be available in memories $EFM^{(i)}$ after the end of filtering.

2. Consider an arbitrary plane z_O. We need to filter and add $\#\Delta lines(z_O)$ into the memories $EFM^{(i)}$. There can be two situations.

   - $\#Lines(z_O + 1) < n_r$. In this case we simply add new filtered rows $\#\Delta lines(z_O)$ into the memories $EFM^{(i)}$.

   - $\#Lines(z_O + 1) \geq n_r$. We need to overwrite some or all previously stored rows because the memory consists of at most n_r rows for each projection. Assume we add some row $y_d \in lines(z_O)$. We store this row using the address $y_d \pmod{n_r}$, and the row, previously stored at this address, will be overwritten. The row with the address y_d and the row with the address $y_d - n_r$ cannot both belong to $lines(z_O)$, because in this case $\#lines(z_O) > n_r$. This is a contradiction.

After the filtering process we will have in memory the filtered detector rows that are in $lines(z_O)$, because

$$\#\Delta lines(z_O) \leq \#lines(z_O) \leq L_{max} \leq n_r.$$

The data, that is overwritten during this process, is not required for the reconstruction of the plane z_O. ☐

4.5.4   Pipelined Reconstruction Schedule

The reconstruction of the volume is performed using the pipelined parallel reconstruction of the planes, contained in the volume. The filtering is performed in parallel to the reconstruction process. Algorithm 10 presents the computation flow.

Before the reconstruction of the upper plane the number $DLCM[0]$ of detector rows is filtered and stored in the memories $EFM^{(i)}$. After this the reconstruction

Algorithm 10 Pipelined Parallel Reconstruction of the Volume

1:	**for** $y_d = 0$ to $DLCM[0] - 1$ **do**	
2:	filter detector row y_d	*(Algorithm 8)*
3:	transfer filtered row into the $EFM^{(i)}$	*(Algorithm 9)*
4:	**end for**	
5:	**for** $z_O = 0$ to $z_{Omax} - 1$ **do**	
6:	reconstruct plane z_O	*(Algorithm 7)*
7:	**if** $z_O < z_{Omax} - 1$ **then**	*(filter data for the next plane)*
8:	**for** $k = 1$ to $DLCM[z_O + 1]$ **do**	
9:	filter row $y_d + k$	*(Algorithm 8)*
10:	transfer filtered data to $EFM^{(i)}$	*(Algorithm 9)*
11:	**end for**	
12:	$y_d \leftarrow y_d + DLCM[z_O + 1]$	*(update the row counter)*
13:	**end if**	
14:	**end for**	

of planes starts. The loop (lines 5-14) goes through all planes sequentially from the upper plane. Two processes are performed in parallel - the reconstruction of a plane (line 6) and the filtering of the detector rows, required for the reconstruction of the next plane (lines 8-12).

The graphical description of these two processes is presented on Figure 4.10(a). By "write" we denote the process when the filtered detector row is transferred into the memories $EFM^{(i)}$ (Algorithm 9). We depicted write phases of the same length. In general the length is variable and the phase might be missing in case when we do not add any new filtered detector row.

Figure 4.10(b) describes the reconstruction of a plane in connection to the filtering process. The geometry computations for the first radial element in a plane are performed during the transfer of the filter data, before the start of the reconstruction itself. The reconstruction of the first radial element in a plane starts when the data transfer if finished and the required filtered data is available.

After the end of the reconstruction of the last radial element in a plane, the data which was filtered during the reconstruction of the current plane, is transferred (Algorithm 9). At the same time the last round of the accumulation is performed.

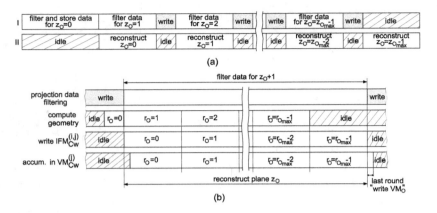

Figure 4.10: Reconstruction of the volume. (a) Pipelining of the two processes. The phase "filter and store data for z_O" contains filtering and transferring the detector rows $y_d \in lines(0)$. (b) Reconstruction of a plane in detail (see Figure 4.8).

4.5.5 Performance Analysis

Modifications of the Cylindrical Algorithm, described in this chapter, accelerate the reconstruction of the volume from cone-beam projections. These modifications are parallelization and pipelining of the backprojection, special scheduling during the reconstruction of the volume.

Table 4.1 presents the information about the main operations, that are performed for the reconstruction of one plane. Obviously, number of operations, required for the reconstruction of the whole volume is obtained multiplying by the number of planes z_{Omax}. No additional operations are required between the reconstruction of two planes. The longest computation is the backprojection, but the number of operations is reduced significantly using b parallel memories, and performing the geometry computations in parallel to the backprojection.

Time required to perform the operations described in Table 4.1 is different for all of these operations. It is implementation specific for each operation. In the next chapter, during the specification of the hardware architecture, we show that during pipelined execution, throughput of the computational modules is one operation

Part	Description of operations	Number of operations
Backprojection of one plane	access to EFM, multiply-accumulate	$\phi_{Omax} \cdot r_{Omax} \cdot p$
Geometry computations	compute intersect points and weighting coefficients	$\phi_{Omax} \cdot r_{Omax}$
Filtering of one row	multiply-accumulate, write into $EIFM$	$N^2 \cdot \phi_{dmax} \cdot DLC[z_O]$
Data transfer	copy from $EIFM$ to EFM	$N \cdot p \cdot DLC[z_O]$

Table 4.1: Main operations, performed for the reconstruction of one plane.

per cycle. Although, multiplication of two operands is performed in three cycles. Another significant reduction of the number of operations is done using the Finite Impulse Response filter. This decreases the number of multiply-accumulate operations to $N \cdot \phi_{dmax}$ for the filtering of each detector row.

4.6 Conclusion

In this section we described the modification of the Cylindrical Algorithm. The parallelization of the backprojection was presented. It was shown that the different computational tasks of the reconstruction can be scheduled in order to minimize the wait time, i.e. when the one task waits for the result of the another task. The implementation of the presented pipelined parallel reconstruction of the volume from the cone-beam projections will be described in the next section.

Chapter 5

Reconstruction Hardware

This section provides the description of the hardware architecture for the reconstruction from cone-beam projections. The hardware architecture is based on the description of the pipelined parallel reconstruction presented in the previous chapter.

5.1 Notation

For the description of the hardware system we use the similar notation as it is defined in [88]:

- for bits $x \in \{0,1\}$ and natural numbers n, we denote by x^n the string consisting of n copies of x, e.g. $0^2 = 00$, $1^4 = 1111$;

- we usually index the bits of strings from right to left with the numbers from 0 to $n-1$

$$a = a_{n-1} \ldots a_0 \in \{0,1\}^n \quad \text{or} \quad a = a[n-1:0];$$

- we denote the natural number with binary representation a as

$$\langle a \rangle = \sum_{i=0}^{n-1} a_i \cdot 2^i \in \{0, \ldots, 2^n - 1\};$$

- fractional numbers are represented as follows:

$$\text{let } a[n-1:0] \in \{0,1\}^n \text{ and } f[1:p-1] \in \{0,1\}^{p-1},$$

101

Name	Width
number of planes z_{Omax}	$z_w = \lceil \log_2 z_{Omax} \rceil$
number of radial elements r_{Omax}	$r_w = \lceil \log_2 r_{Omax} \rceil$
number of voxels ϕ_{Omax}	$\phi_w = \lceil \log_2 \phi_{Omax} \rceil$
detector elements counter	$n = \log_2 N$
width of the control bus for SDRAM	$a_w + 5$
weighting coefficients	wco_w
input projection data	ad_w
filtering coefficients	fk_w
filtered data	af_w
weighted data	aw_w
result of the reconstruction	res_w

Table 5.1: Widths of the design variables and constants.

$$\text{then } \langle a[n-1:0].f[1:p-1]\rangle = \sum_{i=0}^{n-1} a_i \cdot 2^i + \sum_{i=1}^{p-1} f_i \cdot 2^{-i};$$

we permit the cases $p = 0$ and $n = -1$ by defining

$$\langle a.\rangle = \langle a.0\rangle = \langle a\rangle, \ \langle .f\rangle = \langle 0.f\rangle;$$

the obvious identities follow directly

$$\langle 0a.f\rangle = \langle a.f\rangle = \langle a.f0\rangle \text{ and } \langle a.f\rangle = \langle af\rangle \cdot 2^{-(p-1)}.$$

Data Width

Table 5.1 presents the widths of the design constants and variables. The precise values for the variable widths will be introduced in the evaluation of the design.

Basic Circuits

Figure 5.1 denotes the symbols used for gates in drawing circuits. The standard blocks, such as multipliers, dividers, FIFOs, RAMs etc., are depicted with rectangles and have the names MULT, DIV, FIFO and RAM, accordingly. The signal clk denotes the clock signal of the design and the signal $\overline{clk}$ denotes the inverse of this clock. The signal clk is not shown as an input for the environments. Constants

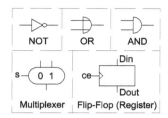

Figure 5.1: Symbols for basic gates.

ϕ_{Omax}, r_{Omax}, z_{Omax} are the design constants and they are not shown as inputs of the environments.

All figures showing circuits are bounded by a dotted rectangle denoting the circuit's *interface*. Signals appearing left of or over the rectangle are *inputs*, right or below – *outputs* of the circuit. Signals, that were named in a figure may be used by their name in other parts of the figure; a single signal can be selected from a bus by the name. A port of the environment can be accessed with the name of the environment module and the port name. For example, the port *Din* of the environment *Aenv* is denoted by the *Aenv.Din*. The abbreviation I/O denotes Input-Output.

Process Flow Description

The architecture consists of several units, each contains a number of environments: circuitry and control. The contents of the circuitry environments are presented using Figures, whereas the control environments will be described by the functional algorithms[1]. This allows to emphasize the functional principles more clearly. In particular, we use the following statements

- the conditional statement:
  if condition **then** {statement 1} **else** {statement 2} **end if**

- the iterative statement: **while** condition **do** statement **end while**

- the **for**-loop:
  for i from ... to ... **do** statement **end for**

---

[1] these algorithms are directly implemented in VHDL

- the **waitfor** statement

    waitfor condition

In the conditional statement (**if**) one of the statements (1 or 2) is executed in the same clock cycle after the condition is checked. In the iterative statements the operations are executed sequentially each clock cycle. When the **waitfor** statement is used, no other operations are performed, until the condition is fulfilled. After the condition is fulfilled, the algorithm continues. If the step size in the **for**-loop is unspecified it is 1 by default.

The notation a^t means the state of the signal a in the cycle t. The notation $a \leftarrow a + 1$ means $a^{t+1} = a^t + 1$. For signals, that are active only one cycle, we use the following notation

$$a^t \leftarrow 0/1/0 \quad \equiv \quad \begin{cases} a^t & \leftarrow 1 \\ a^{t+1} & \leftarrow 0 \end{cases}$$

We ensure that the signal a at cycles t and $t + 1$ is not changed anywhere else.

5.2 Overview of the Architecture

The design, described in this chapter performs all stages of the pipelined parallel reconstruction of the volume from cone-beam projections (part 4). The whole design is placed in one Xilinx FPGA chip, except the memories with the filtered projection data.

We present in this chapter a parametric design, i.e. the values of constants and the bit-widths will be discussed in the evaluation chapter.

5.2.1 Structure

The reconstruction hardware, called a **"3D Backprojector"**, is presented on Figure 5.2 and consists of an FPGA chip and external memory. The reconstruction task is divided into several independent tasks, that are performed by the modules of the design.

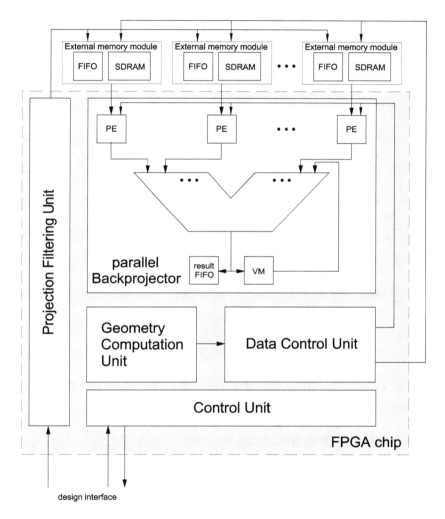

Figure 5.2: Main components of the **3D Backprojector**.

- DESIGN CONTROL The reconstruction of the volume is managed by the Control Unit. All modules of the design are dependent from this unit. It schedules the processes running in the design.

- MEMORY STRUCTURE The filtered projection data is placed in the external (off-chip) memory. Our design supports dynamic memory chips. The high-density FPGA provides enough resources to place all other memories, used during the reconstruction, on-chip.

- PROJECTION FILTERING The detector rows are filtered by the Projection Filtering Unit, and then stored in the external memory using intermediate FIFOs. We use a pipelined implementation of the Finite Impulse Response filter.

- GEOMETRY COMPUTATIONS The computation of the Geometry and the Weighting Coefficients tables are done by the Geometry Computation Unit. The computed values are stored in the Data Control Unit.

- RECONSTRUCTION The Parallel Backprojector, based on the Processing Elements (PEs), performs the reconstruction of the volume. The management of the external memory and the data flow in the Backprojector are done by the Data Control Unit.

5.2.2 Requirements of the Design

Here we describe the requirements and the interface of our design.

Application

The design is developed as a system that consists of one FPGA, FIFO and SDRAM chips. This system must be controlled by the higher level system. During the description we call it an "external device". This can be a PC-based system, connected to the design using one of the standard interfaces[2].

---

[2]the bandwidth of the design is discussed in the evaluation chapter

Preprocessing Conditions

Our design has the following requirements.

- The input projection data must be already pre-weighted with the coefficient (recall definition of p_x and z_y from section 2.8.4)

$$\frac{d \cdot \overline{SO}}{\sqrt{\overline{SO}^2 + p_x^2 + z_y^2}}.$$

In real applications this is done during the logarithmic normalization of the projection data, acquired from the detector using an Analog-Digital Convertor. The values, that are received by the design, are ad_w-bit unsigned integers.

- The design is implemented in FPGA using pre-defined parameters, i.e. it can reconstruct the volume $(z_{Omax}, r_{Omax}, \phi_{Omax})$ from cone-beam projections for some constant values N, d, α, m and $\overline{SO}$ (see description of the Cylindrical Algorithm in section 3.1). The main constants of the design are the following (summarizing from the previous chapters):

  1. the experiment parameters (from section 3.1) are:
     - the half-beam opening angle α,
     - the magnification factor m,
     - the physical size of the detector element d,
     - the distance "X-ray source"-"rotation axis" $\overline{SO}$,
  2. $N = 2^n$ where $n \in \mathbb{Z}^+$,
  3. $r_{Omax} := N/2$,
  4. $\phi_{dmax} = p \cdot b$ where $b, p \in \mathbb{Z}^+$ and p is a power of two,
  5. $\phi_{Omax} := n_\phi \cdot \phi_{dmax}$ where $n_\phi \in \mathbb{Z}_{\geq 1}$,
  6. z_{Omax} is computed using Equation (3.1.15) from section 3.1.7,
  7. n_r is computed using Equation (4.5.1) in section 4.5.1.

- The values of the DLC table, that are computed for the experiment parameter α (section 4.5.1), and the discrete values of the sin() and cos() functions are stored in read-only memories on chip. They are design constants.

- The filter, used in the design, has constant fixed-point coefficients (discrete values of the filter kernel).

Design Interface

The interface of our reconstruction system consists of the following inputs:

- the initialization (reset) signal *rst*,

- the "start reconstruction" signal *gstart*,

- the ad_w-bit bus *PDin* and the "data valid" signal *dwr*,

- the signal *re_vm* used for reading the reconstructed radial element.

The output of the design has the following busses and signals:

- the "filtered data request" signal *drq*,

- the "ready" signal *drdy* for the reconstructed radial element,

- the res_w-bit bus *VMout* used to transfer the result of the reconstruction,

- the signal *rrec* is a "done" signal, activated after the end of the reconstruction of the volume.

Data Transfer

The protocol of the data transfer between the design and the external device is presented on Figures 5.3(a) and (b).

(a) The request of the projection data is initiated by the design using the signal *drq*. The external device transfers the detector row that corresponds to one projection (*N* elements). The detector rows are counted from the upper row

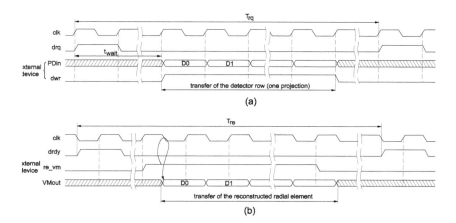

Figure 5.3: Protocol of the data exchange between the design and the external device. (a) Request of the projection data. (b) Download the reconstruction result from the design.

$y_d = 0$ to $N - 1$, and the projections from 0 to $\phi_{d\,max} - 1$. The data are transferred on the bus *PDin* using the "data valid" signal *drw*. The period of the data request

$$T_{rq} := N + TP + T_{wait}$$

clock cycles, where T_{wait} is a number of clock cycles between the request of the data and the activation of the signal *dwr* from the external device, and TP is a number of filtering coefficients (taps). In order to filter N elements a special digital filter (section 5.5.2, Figure 5.11) requires to be cleared (zero-padding). Thus, for the filtering of N elements totaly $N + TP$ cycles are required.

(b) The result of the reconstruction of a radial element is available in the design after the activation of the signal *drdy*. The reconstruction result is computed in two's complement format. The signal *drdy* is activated at the start of the last accumulation round during the reconstruction of each radial element. After this, the external device must activate the signal *re_vm* and hold it for $\phi_{O\,max}$ cycles. The design sends $\phi_{O\,max}$ elements of the reconstructed radial element using the bus *VMout*. These elements are send starting from the element with address $\phi_O = 0$. The radial elements are reconstructed from 0 to $r_{O\,max} - 1$

from the upper plane to the lower. The period of the signal *drdy* is

$$T_{re} > p \cdot \phi_{0max}$$

because of the wait cycles required to operate with the external dynamic memory.

5.2.3 Reconstruction Flow

The design is an implementation of the pipelined parallel reconstruction of the volume from cone-beam projections (see formal description in section 4.5).

The top level control (Algorithm 10) of the reconstruction is provided by the Control Unit. This unit performs the control of the processes running in parallel: the filtering of the projection data, the geometry computations and the reconstruction of a plane. Every process, started by the Control Unit, has an acknowledge ("done") signal on termination.

The filtering is initiated by the Control Unit and is done by the Projection Filtering Unit (Algorithm 8). This unit requests detector data from the external device, filters this data and stores the result of the filtering in the external memory. The transfer of the filtered detector data in the external memory is performed by the Data Control Unit (Algorithm 9).

The calculation of the intersect addresses and the values of the weighting coefficients are done by the Geometry Computation Unit. The result (parts of the Geometry and Weighting Coefficients tables) are stored in the memory of the Data Control Unit.

The reconstruction of the volume is performed in "plane by plane" order. Each plane is processed from the center using the pipelined parallel structure (section 4.3). The reconstruction of the plane is initiated by the Control Unit. The management of the data, required for the reconstruction of a plane, is done by the Data Control Unit. The data from the external memory is received by the processing elements of the Parallel Backprojector. Every processing element weights the input data and reorders it in the corresponding intermediate memory. The summation of the weighted data is performed by the multi-input pipelined adder in the Parallel Backprojector. The result of the reconstruction of each radial element is placed in the result FIFO of the Backprojector. At the end of the reconstruction the signal *rrec* is activated, signaling to the external device that the reconstruction of the whole volume is finished.

5.3 Control Unit

The control logic of the design is combined into the Control Unit. It includes the management of all processes, that are performed during the reconstruction of the volume (described in section 4.5).

Interface

The input signals to the Control Unit are:

- the signal *rst* that is used for initialization of the design,

- the signal *gstart* that is used to initiate the reconstruction process,

- the bus *rdy* that consists of the acknowledge signals from the different modules of the design.

The output signals are:

- the bus *st* contains the start signals for the modules of the design,

- the bus *Y* contains the address of the filtered detector row.

- the output signal *rrec* is a "done" signal for the reconstruction of the whole volume.

Two busses, *st* and *rdy*, are used in the design for the control of the design modules. Table 5.2 shows the components of these busses.

Bus	Component	Purpose	Direction
st	flt	start data filtering	to Projection Filtering Unit
	wr	transfer filtered data	to Data Control Unit
	PE	start reconstruction	to Data Control Unit
	INS	start geometry computations	to Geometry Computation Unit
rdy	flt	filtering is done	from Projection Filtering Unit
	wr	data transfer is done	from Data Control Unit
	PE	reconstruction of the radial element is done	from Data Control Unit

Table 5.2: Control busses of the architecture.

Structure

The Control Unit consists of three environments and one memory. The structure is depicted on Figure 5.4.

- The environment CCenv performs the top-level control of the reconstruction of the whole volume.

- The environment FCCenv is used for the control of the data filtering.

- The environment PECenv controls the Data Control Unit. It activates the reconstruction of a radial element, and initiates the transfer of the filtered data in the external memory.

- The read-only memory DLCM consists of the table DLC.

Computation Flow

The design must be initialized with the signal *rst* before the reconstruction. The reconstruction of the whole volume starts after the signal *gstart* is activated. The reconstruction is performed from the upper plane of the volume. First, the value from the memory $DLCM[0]$ is fetched. This is the number of detector rows, that

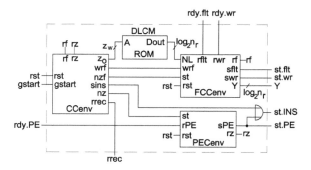

Figure 5.4: Control Unit structure.

are required for the reconstruction of this upper plane (see section 4.5.1). Under the control of the environment FCCenv these detector rows are filtered and stored in the external memories (Algorithms 8 and 9). In parallel to this, the Geometry and Weighting Coefficients tables for the radial element $r_O = 0$ are computed. After $DLCM[0]$ detector rows are filtered, the system is ready for the reconstruction of the first (upper) plane.

The environment CCenv manages two processes during the reconstruction: the backprojection of a plane and the data filtering. This environment generates the control signals to the PECenv and FCCenv. It also processes the signals received from these two environments.

The management of the backprojection is done by the environment PECenv. It includes the scheduling of the backprojection of a plane itself and the computation of the geometry data (intersect addresses and weighting coefficients). When the plane is reconstructed, the environment PECenv signals to the CCenv. After this, the PECenv is ready for the reconstruction of a new plane.

The filtering process is controlled by the environment FCCenv. This environment generates the control signals for the Projection Filtering Unit. The FCCenv receives the number of detector rows ($DLC[z_O]$), that must be filtered and stored in the external memory for the reconstruction of the plane z_O. After one detector row for all projection is filtered, the environment FCCenv waits until the backprojection

113

of a plane is ready, and then copies the filtered data into the external memories. This process (filtering and data transfer) is done $DLC[z_O]$ times. The reconstruction of the new plane starts when the required projection data ($DLC[z_O]$ detector rows) is ready in the external memory (acknowledge from the FCCenv to the CCenv).

After the reconstruction of z_{Omax} planes is done, the signal *rrec* is issued to the external device.

5.3.1 CCenv Environment

The main purpose of this environment is the top-level control of the reconstruction process of the volume. Algorithm 11 describes the management of the reconstruction process. The interface signals of this environment are combined in Table 5.3.

Algorithm 11 CCenv Algorithm

Require: signal *gstart* was issued in the previous cycle

1: $z_O^t \leftarrow 0$	*(start plane)*
2: $sins^t \leftarrow 0/1/0$	*(start geometry computations)*
3: $nzf^{t+1} \leftarrow 0/1/0$	*(start filtering)*
4: $wrf^{t+1} \leftarrow 1$	*(enable data transfer)*
5: **waitfor** $rf = 1$	*(data is ready for the reconstruction)*
6: $wrf \leftarrow 0$	*(disable data transfer)*
7: **for** $z_O = 1$ to z_{Omax} **do**	
8: $\quad nz^t \leftarrow 0/1/0$	*(start reconstruction of plane)*
9: $\quad$ **if** $z_O \neq z_{Omax}$ **then**	
10: $\quad\quad nzf^t \leftarrow 0/1/0$	*(start filtering except the last plane)*
11: $\quad$ **end if**	
12: $\quad$ **waitfor** $rz = 1$	*(end of the plane reconstruction)*
13: $\quad$ **if** $z_O \neq z_{Omax}$ **then**	
14: $\quad\quad wrf \leftarrow 1$	*(enable data transfer)*
15: $\quad\quad$ **waitfor** $rf = 1$	*(filtered data is copied)*
16: $\quad\quad wrf \leftarrow 0$	*(disable data transfer)*
17: $\quad$ **end if**	
18: **end for**	
19: $rrec \leftarrow 0/1/0$	*(reconstruction of the volume is done)*

114

Name	I/O	Width	Purpose
rst	I	1	reset signal
gstart	I	1	global start
rf	I	1	plane filtering "done"
rz	I	1	plane reconstruction "done"
z_O	O	z_w	current plane for filtering
nz	O	1	start reconstruction of a plane
nzf	O	1	start filtering
wrf	O	1	start filtered data transfer
sins	O	1	start geometry computations
rrec	O	1	volume reconstruction "done"

Table 5.3: Interface of the CCenv environment.

The environment is initialized or reset. All internal variables and output control signals are cleared.

1: **if** $rst = 1$ **then**

2:    $z_O \leftarrow 0, nz \leftarrow 0, nzf \leftarrow 0, wrf \leftarrow 0, sins \leftarrow 0, rrec \leftarrow 0$

3: **end if**

When the input signal *gstart* is activated by the external device, the reconstruction of the volume begins with the preparation phase (lines 1-4). This is a processing of data, required for the reconstruction of the upper plane. The detector rows required for the reconstruction of the first plane are filtered and stored in the external memory under the management of the environment FCCenv (start signal nzf). The data transfer is enabled from the beginning ($wrf^{t+1} \leftarrow 1$) in order to perform the non-stop filtering and transfer of the filtered rows.

In parallel to filtering, the geometry computations for the first radial element of the upper plane are performed. They are initiated by the signal *sins*.

After all required data for the reconstruction of the upper plane is ready, the main loop starts (lines 7-18). The loop counter goes from 1 to z_{Omax} instead of 0 to $z_{Omax} - 1$ because it is used only as an address of the memory *DLCM*. The projection data for plane z_O is filtered during the backprojection of the plane $z_O - 1$ (see pipelined reconstruction schedule in section 4.5.4). The reconstruction of plane

$z_O - 1$ is started by activating signal nz (line 8). After this, the CCenv waits for the end of the reconstruction of a plane (signal rz), and then activates the transfer of the filtered data ($wrf \leftarrow 1$). When the index z_O is equal to the maximum value z_{Omax} the filtering is not performed[3] (lines 9-11 and 13-17). The signal $rrec$ is issued to the external device at the end of the reconstruction of the whole volume.

5.3.2 FCCenv Environment

The environment FCCenv performs the control of the data filtering, which is done by the Projection Filtering Unit (see description in section 5.5). The control of the filtering is described by Algorithm 12. The interface signals are shown in Table 5.4.

Algorithm 12 FCCenv Algorithm

Require: signal st was issued in the previous cycle

1: **if** $NL \neq 0$ **then**   *(check if nothing is to filter for this plane)*
2:    $ycnt \leftarrow 1$
3:    **while** $ycnt \leq NL$ **do**   *(filter all lines that are in $\Delta lines(z_O)$)*
4:      $sflt \leftarrow 0/1/0$ *(start filter)*
5:      **waitfor** $rflt = 1$ *(end of the filtering of the row)*
6:      **waitfor** $wrf = 1$ *(enable data transfer from CCenv)*
7:      $swr \leftarrow 1$ *(start data transfer)*
8:      **waitfor** $rwr = 1$ *(data transfer "done")*
9:      $swr \leftarrow 0$ *(stop data transfer)*
10:     $Y \leftarrow Y + 1 \,(\mathrm{mod}\ n_r), ycnt \leftarrow ycnt + 1$
11:    **end while**
12: **else**   *(NL = 0, wait for the activation of wrf)*
13:    **waitfor** $wrf = 1$
14: **end if**
15: $rf^t \leftarrow 0/1/0$ *(filtering is done)*

For the reconstruction of a plane z_O a number of detector rows must be filtered (recall the definition of the table DLC from section 4.5.1). This number of rows is fetched from memory DLCM using address $z_O[z_w - 1 : 0]$ and is received by environment FCCenv on port NL (see Figure 5.4).

---
[3] see Figure 4.10(a)

116

Name	I/O	Width	Purpose
rst	I	1	reset signal
st	I	1	start signal
NL	I	$\log_2 n_r$	input value $DLCM[z_O]$
wrf	I	1	enable transfer of the filtered data
rflt	I	1	row filtering "done"
rwr	I	1	data transfer "done"
rf	O	1	plane filtering "done"
sflt	O	1	start row filtering
swr	O	1	start data transfer
Y	O	$\log_2 n_r$	current detector row

Table 5.4: Interface of the FCCenv environment.

After the signal st is activated by the CCenv (signal nzf), environment FCCenv starts. It controls the filtering of NL detector rows. This is a two stage process for each row. First, the row is filtered for all projections (lines 4-5) (this is done by the Projection Filtering Unit). Second, this filtered row is transferred into the memories $EFM^{(i)}$ from the memories $EIFM^{(i)}$ (lines 6-9) (this is done by the Data Control Unit). The data is written into $EFM^{(i)}$ using row address Y. After the data is transferred, the next detector row is filtered if $NL > 1$.

During the reconstruction of plane z_O the filtering is performed for the plane $z_O + 1$ (see Figures 4.10 and 5.5). When the detector row is filtered we wait until the end of the reconstruction of the plane (line 6), because the external memories with the filtered projection data are busy during this process and we cannot write the new filtered data. This new filtered projection data is transferred after the reconstruction of the plane is complete (lines 7-9). If $NL > 1$ (see Figure 5.5(b)) we filter and transfer data for the next detector row etc. until NL rows are ready. This process is performed now without additional waiting (line 6), because the signal wrf stays active (lines 14-15 in Algorithm 11). After all required rows are filtered, the environment sends the signal rf to the CCenv.

If $NL = 0$, i.e. there is nothing to filter for the next plane, we simply wait (line 13) until the signal wrf is activated by the CCenv.

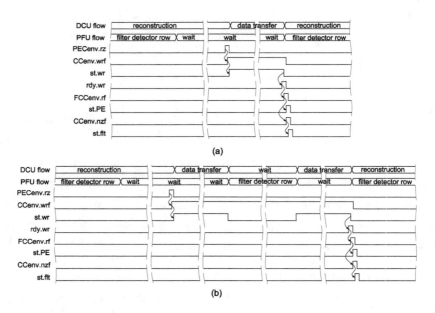

Figure 5.5: Two processes running in parallel: reconstruction and filtering detector rows. (a) $DLC[z_O] = 1$. (b) $DLC[z_O] = 2$. Abbreviations: "DCU" is the Data Control Unit, and "PFU" is the Projection Filtering Unit.

118

Name	I/O	Width	Purpose
rst	I	1	reset signal
st	I	1	start signal
rPE	I	1	radial element reconstruction "done"
rz	O	1	plane reconstruction "done"
sPE	O	1	start radial element reconstruction

Table 5.5: Interface of the PECenv environment.

The variables and output signals are initialized on reset.

1: **if** $rst = 1$ **then**

2:     $sflt \leftarrow 0,\ swr \leftarrow 0,\ rf \leftarrow 0,\ Y \leftarrow 0$

3: **end if**

5.3.3 PECenv Environment

The reconstruction of the plane is performed under the high-level control of the environment PECenv (Algorithm 13). Table 5.5 shows the input and output signals of this environment.

Algorithm 13 PECenv Algorithm

Require: signal st was active in the previous cycle

1: **for** $r_O = 0$ to $r_{Omax} - 1$ **do**

2:     $sPE^t \leftarrow 0/1/0$ *(start reconstruction of the radial element)*

3:     **waitfor** $rPE = 1$ *(end of the reconstruction of the radial element)*

4: **end for**

5: $rz^t \leftarrow 0/1/0$ *(plane reconstruction is done)*

The environment PECenv is initialized on reset:

1: **if** $rst = 1$ **then**

2:     $sPE \leftarrow 0,\ rz \leftarrow 0,\ r_O \leftarrow 0.$

3: **end if**

The environment PECenv starts when the signal st is activated by the CCenv (signal nz). It sends the signal sPE to the Data Control Unit to initiate the reconstruction of a radial element. The same signal is used to start the Geometry Com-

119

putations Unit for next radial element (see Figure 5.4). The environment PECenv waits until the end of the reconstruction of a radial element[4] (line 3). When the radial element is reconstructed, the Data Control Unit activates the signal $rdy.PE$, which is connected to the input rPE of the PECenv. After r_{Omax} radial elements are reconstructed, the signal rz is sent to the environment CCenv and the reconstruction of a plane is finished.

5.4 Memory Subsystem

Due to the large size of the filtered data required for the reconstruction it cannot be placed in the RAM inside the FPGA chip. Thus, an external memory structure is required.

5.4.1 Selection of the Memory Type

The amount of filtered data, that must be stored for the reconstruction of an arbitrary plane can be estimated as follows. For the reconstruction of one plane $N \cdot n_r \cdot \phi_{dmax}$ filtered elements must be stored. Taking the following parameters: $N = 512$, $n_r = 64$, $\phi_{dmax} = 384$ and the width of the elements $af_w = 16$ bit, we obtain that the whole memory with the filtered projection data has the capacity of 24 MBytes. This amount of data must be placed outside the FPGA chip. Comparing static and dynamic random-access memories (SRAMs and SDRAMs), the usage of dynamic RAM keeps the price of the system reasonable for such amount of data. The usage of SDRAM simplifies the scale of our hardware system for the greater problems, e.g. with $N = 1024$ and higher[5].

We will describe the memory subsystem based on dynamic memory. The corresponding module - Data Control Unit, supports all the required operations for dynamic memory. In case of using static memory the Data Control Unit can be simplified.

---

[4]the geometry computations are always faster than the reconstruction of a radial element; thus we wait until the end of the reconstruction

[5]using detectors with a greater number of elements

Dynamic memory is organized as a cell array with rows and columns. Each memory chip consists of multiple cell arrays that are called banks. An access to the data in the SDRAM chip consists of a row access with the row address strobe signal (RAS) and the bank address (BA). The opening of a row is followed by the column address with the column address strobe signal (CAS). The consistency of data in dynamic memory is provided by the periodic access to all memory cells, i.e. performing refresh of the memory.

We describe the design with SDRAM chips, which have the following structure. The chip contains two internal banks (bank select signal BA), each bank has n_r rows and each row has 2^{n-1} elements (columns). For the simplicity of the description, we treat the input and output of SDRAM chip as two separate busses with equal width[6]. The sequences of commands, e.g. activating/deactivating a bank, are descriptive, i.e. showing only the logic sequence of operations.

5.4.2 External Memory Structure

The external memory structure is used to store the filtered projection data. The memories of this structure were defined during the formal description in section 4.5.2.

Structure

There are b modules in the external memory structure (see Figure 5.6). They are connected to the common busses: the address bus CA, the input data bus $FDin$ and the control bus CF. Each module has it's own output data bus. Figure 5.7 presents the structure of one module. The memory $EFM^{(i)}$, defined in section 4.2.2, is implemented as a SDRAM chip, and the intermediate memory $EIFM^{(i)}$, defined in section 4.5.2, is a FIFO.

---

[6]normally, SDRAM chips have bidirectional data bus

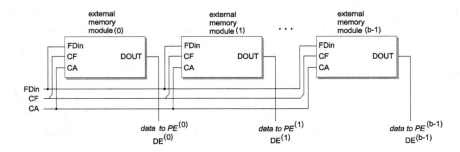

Figure 5.6: Connection of the external memory modules.

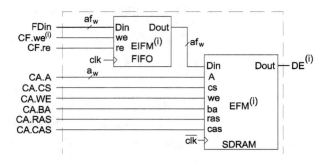

Figure 5.7: Internal structure of the ith external memory module.

Memory Module Interface

The FIFOs in the external memory modules have the common af_w-bit input data bus $FDin$ and they are controlled using the bus CF. This bus consists of:

- the FIFO "write enable" signals $we^{(i)}$ $i \in [0 : b - 1]_{\mathbb{Z}}$,

- the FIFO "read enable" signal re.

Each signal $CF.we^{(i)}$ is connected to the corresponding i^{th} FIFO. The "read enable" signal $CF.re$ is connected to all FIFO chips.

The SDRAM chips are controlled by the bus CA. This bus consists of the following signals:

- the a_w-bit wide address bus $A[a_w - 1 : 0]$,

- the signal "bank address" BA,

- the signal "chip select" CS,

- the signal "write enable" WE,

- the signal "row address" RAS,

- the signal "column address" CAS.

The common control bus CA allows to operate with all b SDRAM chips in parallel, accessing, writing and refreshing them simultaneously. This simplifies the data management of the memory system.

Each ith external memory module has an af_w-bit output data bus $DE^{(i)}$, which is an output of the ith SDRAM chip.

Internal Data Storage

The filtered projection memory $EFM^{(i)}$ from the section 4.5.2 is mapped into the SDRAM chip as follows (see graphical description on Figure 5.8). Recall that the number of projections is $\phi_{d\,max} = p \cdot b$, and that n_r is a maximum number of detector

123

rows, required for the reconstruction of a plane. We describe the allocation of the filtered data in the SDRAM chip for the case, when one row in one internal bank consists of $N/2$ columns. For the case of bigger N, the appropriate memory chip must be selected, e.g. with the higher number of internal banks.

- The index of the module, that contains the projection i_ϕ is defined as

$$i := \lfloor i_\phi/p \rfloor \, .$$

- The address of the element $[x_d, y_d, i_\phi]$ inside this module is computed as follows. The internal bank, that contains this element is

$$A_b := \lfloor 2 \cdot x_d/N \rfloor .$$

The address of the element $[x_d, y_d, i_\phi]$ inside the bank A_b for is (for $i_\phi \in [0 : \phi_{d\,max} - 1]_\mathbb{Z}$):

$$A := N \cdot n_r \cdot A_p + N \cdot A_r + A_o \qquad (5.4.1)$$

where

$$A_p := i_\phi \ (\mathrm{mod}\ p) \qquad\qquad (projection\ address)$$
$$A_r := y_d \ (\mathrm{mod}\ n_r) \qquad\qquad (row\ address)$$
$$A_o := x_d \ (\mathrm{mod}\ (N/2)) \qquad\qquad (offset\ inside\ the\ row\ A_r)$$

The usage of the external memory is described in section 5.7 where the interface of the design to the SDRAMs is presented.

5.5 Projection Filtering Unit

The data from the detector, required for the reconstruction of the volume is received and processed in the Projection Filtering Unit. This unit is controlled by the environment FCCenv of the Control Unit.

Interface

The filtering is initialized by the Control Unit using the input signal $st.flt$. The adw-bit input bus $PDin$ transfers the projection data into the environment, which

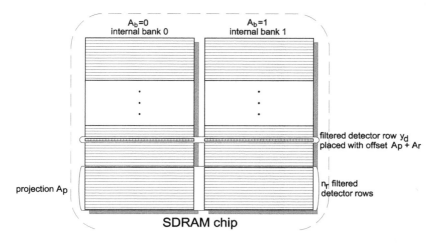

Figure 5.8: Filtered data allocation in the SDRAM chip. Every row in each bank has $N/2$ elements

performs the convolution of the input data with the filtering kernel. The signal *dwr* is activated when the data on the bus *PDin* is available. The design signal *rst* is used for the initialization of the unit.

The af_w-bit output bus *FDin* transfers the filtered values into the FIFOs of the external memory structure. Output bus *CF* consists of "write enable" signals for the external FIFOs (control signals signals are "active low"). Output signal *drq* is used to request a detector row for filtering from the external device. Output signal *rdy.flt* is an acknowledge for the Control Unit when the filtering of the detector row is done.

Structure

The structure of the Projection Filtering Unit is presented on Figure 5.9.

- The filtering process is controlled by the environment FDenv. It generates the request for the new projection data, and controls the write of the filtered values into the FIFOs of the external memory.

- Environment FLTenv is a pipelined filter. It is an implementation of the convolution of the input projection values with the filter kernel.

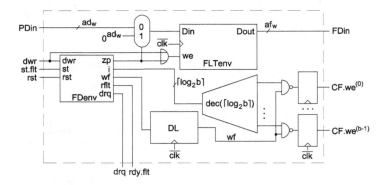

Figure 5.9: Structure of the Projection Filtering Unit.

- The delay line DL compensates the pipelined delay of the FLTenv for the output "write enable" signal.

- The decoder $dec()$ processes the binary value of the projection group counter in order to select the external memory module to store the filtered values.

Computation Flow

The filtering of the projection data is performed in the following order: the detector row is filtered for all projections from 0 to $\phi_{dmax} - 1$ sequentially. The filtering process is initiated by the activation of the input signal $st.flt$ from the FCCenv in the Control Unit. After this, the signal drq is activated signaling for the external device that the new detector row is waited. The projection values are received by the FLTenv using the bus $PDin$. The signal dwr is active when the data is transferred on the bus $PDin$ (refer to Figure 5.3(a) in the description of the design interface in section 5.2.2).

Environment FLTenv has a pipelined structure for the data filtering. It implements the symmetric Finite Impulse Response (FIR) filter with a pre-defined number of coefficients (taps). This number is a design constant TP. The data load into the FLTenv can be initiated either by the external device using the signal dwr, or by the FDenv using the signal zp. The FDenv controls the data input into the FLTenv in

126

such a way, that the filter pipeline is cleared after the filtering of each detector row (zero-padding technique). The FLTenv outputs the signed filtered values in two's complement format because the filtering kernel has positive and negative values. The filtered values belong to the interval $[-2^{af_w-1} : 2^{af_w-1} - 1]_{\mathbb{Z}}$. The output of the FLTenv is connected to the bus $FDin$ which is common for all FIFOs of the external memory structure. The output "write enable" signal wf from the environment FDenv is active when the FLTenv performs filtering. This signal is delayed for the time of the pipeline delay of the filtered data output. After p projections of one detector row are filtered and saved into one FIFO $EIFM^{(i)}$, the index i of the projection group is incremented and the next external memory module is selected.

5.5.1 FDenv Environment

The control of the filtering unit FLTenv is provided by environment FDenv. Algorithm 14 specifies the filtering control.

Algorithm 14 FDenv Algorithm

Require: signal st was issued in the previous cycle

1: $drq^t \leftarrow 0/1/0$ (*request data from the external device*)
2: **waitfor** $dwr = 1$ (*wait for the first input projection data*)
3: $wf \leftarrow 1$ (*enable output write signal*)
4: **waitfor** $dwr = 0$ (*end of the input data*)
5: $wf \leftarrow 0$ (*disable output write signal*)
6: $\langle$ clear the pipe in FLTenv $\rangle$
7: $i_p^t \leftarrow i_p^{t-1} + 1$ (*counter of the projections in a group*)
8: **if** $i_p = p$ **then**
9:     $i_p^t \leftarrow 0$ (*reset the counter*)
10:     $i^t \leftarrow i^{t-1} + 1$
11:     **if** $i = b$ **then**
12:         $i^t \leftarrow 0$ (*reset the group counter*)
13:     **end if**
14: **end if**
15: $rflt^t \leftarrow 0/1/0$ (*row filtering is done*)

When the FDenv is started (signal $st.flt$) it requests N elements from the external device, that provides the projection data. The time between the request of the data

($drq = 1$) and the arriving of the data ($dwr = 1$) is the waiting time (t_{wait}). This parameter is used in the analysis of the implementation. The signal wf is activated (line 3) when the data is available ($drw = 1$). After all N elements are loaded into the FLTenv, the input signal dwr is deactivated (line 4). This is a condition to stop writing the output elements. It is done by setting the signal wf to zero (line 5). The signal wf is delayed (see Figure 5.9) by the delay line in order to align the "write enable" signal $CF.we^{(i)}$ to the output of the FLTenv.

When the filtering is done, we reset the environment FLTenv as follows.

$\langle$ clear the pipe in FLTenv $\rangle \equiv$

1: **for** $k = 0$ to TP **do**

2: $\quad zp \leftarrow 1$ $\qquad\qquad\qquad\qquad\qquad$ (*write $TP + 1$ zeros into the FLTenv*)

3: **end for**

4: $zp \leftarrow 0$

This process is called zero-padding [89]. After the pipe in the FLTenv is cleared, the new data can be processed. We increment the counter of the projections i_p in one group of p projections. When this counter is equal to p, we reset it and increment the counter of the groups of projections i (line 10). The binary value of this counter is decoded, and the corresponding signal after the decoder selects the external memory module (see Figure 5.9). This counter is cleared when it's value is equal to b, i.e. the detector row for all projections $\phi_{dmax} = p \cdot b$ was filtered. The acknowledge signal $rflt$ is send to the Control Unit after the filtering of each N elements (one detector row).

On reset the following sequence is executed

1: **if** $rst = 1$ **then**

2: $\quad i \leftarrow 0, i_p \leftarrow 0$ $\qquad\qquad\qquad\qquad\qquad\qquad$ (*reset the counters*)

3: $\quad rflt \leftarrow 0, wf \leftarrow 0, drq \leftarrow 0$

4: $\quad \langle$ clear the pipe in FLTenv $\rangle$

5: **end if**

5.5.2   FLTenv Environment

The discrete convolution of the projection data and the filter kernel (see section 2.8.2) is done by the environment FLTenv. This environment is a direct implementation of the FIR filter [89] with the coefficients that are pre-defined during the design[7]. The number of filtering coefficients is denoted by TP and can be up to N. The filtering described by (2.8.2) can be rewritten now as

$$W_d(x_d, i_\phi) = d \sum_{k=-(TP-1)}^{TP-1} P_d(x_d - k, i_\phi) \cdot h(kd) \quad \forall x_d \in [0 : N-1]_{\mathbb{Z}},$$

where the function P_d is zero for all $(x_d - k) \notin [0 : N-1]_{\mathbb{Z}}$. This condition means, that we have to insert TP zeros between any two sets of N data values, i.e. one detector row for one projection. Thus, we have $(N + TP)$ cycles for filtering of N values. The number of taps also defines the period of data request for filtering $T_{rq} := N + TP + T_{wait}$. The multiplication by d is included into the weighting of the input projection data (see pre-processing conditions in section 5.2.2). Obviously, the number of taps influences the quality of filtering. The discussion is presented in section 6.3.

The FIR structure is shown on Figure 5.10. As the implementation of the FIR filter we used a highly optimized IP Core from the Xilinx Core Generator system, which employ no multipliers in the design, but only Look-Up Tables (LUTs), shift registers and an accumulator [90]. The selection of the IP Core from Xilinx is made only for efficiency reasons.

The interface of the FLTenv consists of:

- the input bus *Din* for the values of the detector elements,

- the input signal *we* is used to load the values on the bus *Din*,

- the output bus *Dout* is used to transfer the filtered values from the FLTenv. The values on this bus are numbers in two's complement format.

---

[7]Xilinx FIR IP Core can be configured to load new filter coefficients

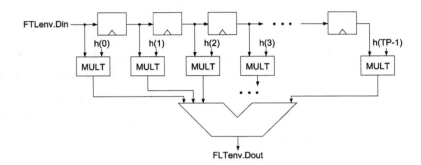

Figure 5.10: Block diagram of the FIR filter in the FLTenv. Function $h()$ is a kernel of the filter.

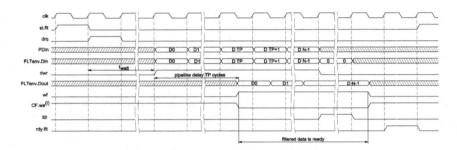

Figure 5.11: Timing Diagram. Filtering.

Figure 5.11 presents the timing diagram of the Projection Filtering Unit. The elements of the detector row are received by the filter FLTenv through the input bus *Din* under the control of signal *we* (Figure 5.9). The circuitry of the FLTenv is clocked with the signal $\overline{clk}$. After $(TP + 1)$ clock signals the filtered values are available on the output bus *Dout* of the FLTenv which is connected to the bus *FDin*. The filtered values are stored in the FIFOs $EIFM^{(i)}$ of the external memory structure.

The width of the output filtered data is obtained as follows [91]. The input data is ad_w-bit wide unsigned integers. The coefficients of the filtering function are signed values. They are normalized, and belong to the interval $[-1, 1]$. We represent them as signed fixed-point numbers with fk_w-bit fractional part. The products of the input data with the filtering kernel are signed $(ad_w + fk_w)$-bit numbers. There are TP such products, that are accumulated together. The result is $(ad_w + fk_w + tp_w)$-bit signed number

$$af_w := ad_w + fk_w + tp_w$$

where $tp_w := \lceil \log_2 TP \rceil$. For the case of constant filter coefficients, the Xilinx FIR IP Core is optimized to reduce the number of output bits [91].

5.6 Geometry Computation Unit

The Geometry and Weighting Coefficients tables are computed in parallel to the backprojection process and stored in the on-chip memory. In this section we describe the the whole process of the geometry computations.

5.6.1 Geometry Computations

For the hardware implementation, Algorithm 4 and the equations from section 3.1.7 must be optimized. As it was described, the computation of the Geometry Table (with the values of the ray-detector intersection addresses) has two independent terms: horizontal and vertical intersection coordinates (Equations (3.1.11) and (3.1.16)). In the hardware implementation one part from these equations is calculated for both terms.

Transformation

Recall the Equation (3.1.17) from section 3.1.7 for the Geometry Table

$$
\begin{aligned}
INS[z_O, r_O, \phi_O] &= z_d \cdot N + p_d \\
&= \frac{N}{d} \cdot \frac{\overline{SO} \cdot m \cdot (z_O - z_{Omax}/2) \cdot \Delta z_O}{\overline{SO} - r_{Oa} \cdot \cos(\phi_{Oa})} + N \cdot \left(\frac{N}{2} - 1\right) \\
&\quad + \frac{1}{d} \cdot \frac{\overline{SO} \cdot m \cdot r_{Oa} \cdot \sin(\phi_{Oa})}{\overline{SO} - r_{Oa} \cdot \cos(\phi_{Oa})} + \frac{N}{2} - 1.
\end{aligned}
$$

Basing on the definitions of variables Δr_O and R_{max} from section 3.1.7, we make the following simplification

$$\Delta r_O \cdot \frac{m}{d} = \frac{2 \cdot R_{max}}{2 \cdot r_{Omax} - 1} \cdot \frac{m}{d}$$
$$= \frac{2 \cdot N \cdot d \cdot \cos(\alpha)}{2 \cdot m(2 \cdot r_{Omax} - 1)} \cdot \frac{m}{d}$$
$$= \frac{N \cdot \cos(\alpha)}{2 \cdot r_{Omax} - 1}.$$

We use the definitions of $r_{Oa} := \Delta r_O \cdot r_O$ and $\Delta z_O := \Delta r_O$ from section 3.1.7, and set $z_c := z_O - \lfloor z_{Omax}/2 \rfloor$. Henceforth we compute value $z_{Omax}/2$ rounded down because we use only integer (fixed-point) values during the computations. We transform and regroup terms in the equation for $INS[z_O, r_O, \phi_O]$ as follows

$$INS[z_O, r_O, \phi_O] = N \cdot z_c \cdot \frac{\Delta r_O \cdot m/d}{1 - r_O \cdot \cos(\phi_{Oa}) \cdot \Delta r_O / \overline{SO}} + N \cdot (\frac{N}{2} - 1)$$
$$+ r_O \cdot \sin(\phi_{Oa}) \cdot \frac{\Delta r_O \cdot m/d}{1 - r_O \cdot \cos(\phi_{Oa}) \cdot \Delta r_O / \overline{SO}} + \frac{N}{2} - 1,$$
$$= N \cdot z_c \cdot C(r_O, \phi_O) + N \cdot (\frac{N}{2} - 1)$$
$$+ r_O \cdot \sin(\phi_{Oa}) \cdot C(r_O, \phi_O) + \frac{N}{2} - 1,$$

where

$$C(r_O, \phi_O) = \frac{N \cdot \cos(\alpha)/(2 \cdot r_{Omax} - 1)}{1 - r_O \cdot \cos(\phi_{Oa}) \cdot \Delta r_O / \overline{SO}} \tag{5.6.1}$$

is a "common term".

Calculation of the Intersect Address

Using this transformation the computation of each intersection coordinate for the voxel (z_O, r_O, ϕ_O) has several stages.

1. Compute the value $C(r_O, \phi_O)$.

2. Compute the horizontal coordinate

$$p_d = r_O \cdot \sin(\phi_{Oa}) \cdot C(r_O, \phi_O) + N/2 - 1. \tag{5.6.2}$$

3. Compute the vertical coordinate

$$z_d = z_c \cdot C(r_O, \phi_O) + N/2 - 1 \quad (\text{mod } n_r). \qquad (5.6.3)$$

From now on we compute the coordinate z_d modulo n_r because during the reconstruction of a plane we work with maximum n_r filtered detector rows (recall the description of the projection of a plane in section 4.5.1).

4. Obtain the intersect value $N \cdot z_d + p_d$. This is a $(\log_2 n_r + n)$-bit wide value.

All fractional parts of the variables in presented formulas are truncated during the conversion to the integer values. This simplifies the hardware implementation.

Calculation of the Weighting Coefficients

In order to calculate the value of the elements of the Weighting Table the computation of the "common term" can be used partially. Recall the definition of the Weighting Table (section 3.1.8):

$$WT[r_O, \phi_O] = \frac{\overline{SO}^2}{(\overline{SO} - r_{Oa} \cdot \cos(\phi_{Oa}))^2}.$$

Using the above introduced reordering, obtain:

$$WT[r_O, \phi_O] = \frac{1}{(1 - r_O \cdot \cos(\phi_{Oa}) \cdot \Delta r_O / \overline{SO})^2}. \qquad (5.6.4)$$

5.6.2 Variables and Constants

For the real square detector, e.g. with parameters $d = 0.4$mm and $N = 512$, we limit the half-beam opening angle α to the interval $[2.5°, 7.5°]$. We introduce the constants and variables of the computations and define the range of each variable[8]:

- $Na := N \cdot \cos(\alpha)/(2r_{Omax} - 1)$, $Na \in (0, 2)$

- $SORc := \Delta r_O / \overline{SO}$, $SORc \in (0, 1)$

- $CW := 1/(1 - r_O \cdot \cos(\phi_{Oa}) \cdot SORc)$, $CW \in (0, 2)$

---

[8]Using the above mentioned parameters we computed the values of the constants and variables (Na, $SORc$, CW and CW^2) for the values $\alpha \in [2.5°, 7.5°]$. The result of the computations defined the bounds of these constants and variables.

- $CW^2 < 2$ and $CW \cdot Na < 2$

The constants of the design have the following representation[9]:

1. the constant Na is an unsigned fixed point number

$$\langle Na[na_w : 0] \rangle \cdot 2^{-na_w},$$

2. the constant $SORc$ is an unsigned fixed point number

$$\langle SORc[s_w - 1 : 0] \rangle \cdot 2^{-s_w},$$

3. the values of the transcendental functions are stored in tables in the following way. The ϕ_{Omax} many values of the transcendental functions correspond to the whole period 2π (recall that $\Delta\phi := 2\pi/\phi_{Omax}$ in section 3.1.7). These values are unsigned fixed-point numbers that belong to the interval $[0, 1]$:

$$\langle sint[si_w : 0] \rangle \cdot 2^{-si_w} \text{ and } \langle cost[co_w : 0] \rangle \cdot 2^{-co_w}.$$

The signs $sneg$ for the sin() and $cneg$ for the cos() functions are computed using the value of the voxel counter ϕ_O

$$sneg = \begin{cases} 0 & \text{if } \phi_O \in [0, 0.5 \cdot \phi_{Omax}] \\ 1 & \text{if } \phi_O \in [0.5 \cdot \phi_{Omax} + 1, \phi_{Omax} - 1] \end{cases} \quad (5.6.5)$$

$$cneg = \begin{cases} 0 & \text{if } \phi_O \in [0, 0.25 \cdot \phi_{Omax}] \cup [0.75 \cdot \phi_{Omax}, \phi_{Omax} - 1] \\ 1 & \text{if } \phi_O \in [0.25 \cdot \phi_{Omax} + 1, 0.75 \cdot \phi_{Omax} - 1] \end{cases}.$$

The output values of the geometry computations have the following representation:

- the intersect coordinate is an unsigned integer number

$$\langle ins[n + \log_2 n_r - 1 : 0] \rangle,$$

- the weighting coefficient $wcoe \in (0, 2)$ is an unsigned fixed-point number

$$\langle wcoe[wco_w : 0] \rangle \cdot 2^{-wco_w}.$$

---

[9]recall that $N = 2^n$

5.6.3 Architecture Overview

The Geometry Computations Unit is controlled by the environment PECenv of the Control Unit. It performs the calculation of the intersection addresses and the weighting coefficients for one radial element.

Interface

The input signals of the Geometry Computation Unit are:

- the signal $st.INS$ that is used to start the geometry computations,

- the signal rst that is used for the initialization.

The output of the Geometry Computation Unit contains the following busses and signals:

- the data busses $ins[n + \log_2 n_r - 1 : 0]$ and $wcoe[wco_w : 0]$ that are used for the intersection address and weighting coefficient values accordingly;

- the signals we_ins and we_wc are "data valid" signals. They correspond to the busses ins and $wcoe$.

Structure

The geometry computations are carried out in a specialized structure presented on Figure 5.12. It consists of the following environments:

- the environment INSCenv is used for generation of counters ϕ_O, r_O, z_O and for the control of the whole flow of the geometry computations,

- the environment TSCenv provides values of the transcendental functions and their signs,

- the environment COMTenv performs the computation of the "common term" value,

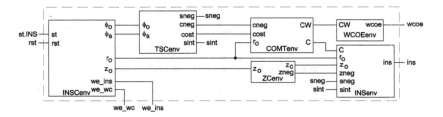

Figure 5.12: Geometry computation unit.

- the environment ZCenv computes the plane shift relative to the center of the volume[10],

- the environment WCOEenv computes the weighting coefficients,

- the environment INSenv calculates values of the intersection coordinates.

Computation Flow

The Geometry Computation Unit calculates the following values: the intersection addresses and the weighting coefficients. These values are computed for the voxels of the particular radial element in the plane. Computations are fully pipelined: each standard arithmetic module has a particular number of stages.

The environment INSCenv performs the scheduling of the computations using the control signals. It receives the start signal and begins to generate the counter ϕ_O. Data from the table $cost()$ fetched using this counter (TSCenv) is send to the environment COMTenv. This environment is used for the computation of the "common term". The signs of the sin() and cos() functions (5.6.5) are computed using the value of the counter ϕ_O and the constants in the environment TSCenv. As the computation of the "common term" is pipelined, the fetch of the sin() value and the computation of it's sign are delayed. This is done in the INSCenv using delay lines and a special counter.

---

[10]i.e. $z_c := z_O - \lfloor z_{Omax}/2 \rfloor$

136

The environment COMTenv provides the "common term" for the two environments - WCOEenv and INSenv. The WCOEenv computes the weighting coefficients, and outputs these values using the bus *wcoe*.

The INSenv computes the intersect address value using the input data from different environments: the "common term" from the COMTenv and the value of the plane counter from the ZCenv. The environment INSenv uses the values of the sin() function with the sign *sneg*. The output of the INSenv is the value of the intersection coordinate, combined from the vertical and horizontal intersection coordinates. The values of the intersection coordinates are available on the output bus *ins*. The signals *we_ins* and *we_wc* are active when the output busses (*ins* and *wcoe*) contain the valid data.

The geometry computations for one radial element are performed faster than the backprojection of one radial element. Therefore, no acknowledge for the Control Unit is required after the end of the geometry computations.

5.6.4 Control Environment INSCenv

The whole geometry computation process is controlled by the INSCenv. This environment generates the signals and counters required for the computations in the Geometry Computation Unit.

Interface

The input interface of the INSCenv consist of two control signals: start signal (*st*) and initialization signal (*rst*). The output of the INSCenv has the following signals:

- the bus $z_O[z_w - 1 : 0]$ is used to transfer the values of the plane counter,

- the bus $r_O[r_w - 1 : 0]$ is used to transfer the values of radial elements counter,

- the busses $\phi_O[\phi_w - 1 : 0]$ and $\phi_S[\phi_w - 1 : 0]$ are used to transfer the non-delayed and delayed values of the voxels counter respectively,

- the signals *we_wc* and *we_ins* are "data valid" signals for the outputs of the Geometry Computation Unit.

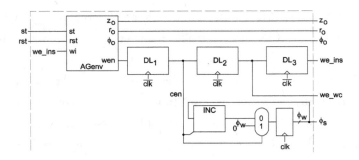

Figure 5.13: Structure of the INSCenv.

Structure and Data Flow

The internal structure of the INSCenv is shown on Figure 5.13. Environment IN-SCenv consists of environment AGenv, delay lines and a special counter, based on the incrementor.

The counters (z_O, r_O, ϕ_O) are generated by the AGenv. The values of these counters are used by other environments in the Geometry Computations Unit. Environment AGenv outputs also a control signal, namely *wen*. This signal is delayed by the three delay lines (DL_1, DL_2 and DL_3). These delay lines are implemented as shift registers.

First delay line DL_1 compensates the delay of the logic, contained in the COMTenv. The output of the delay line (signal *cen*) is used to generate the values of the delayed counter ϕ_O for the table $sint()$ in TSCenv. The values are generated using the incrementor and are stored in the intermediate register. The delayed values are available on the output bus $\phi_S[\phi_w - 1 : 0]$. Whereas signal *wen* (and the signal *cen* respectively) stays active only ϕ_{Omax} many clock cycles (see Algorithm 15), the generated values ϕ_S belong to the interval $[0 : \phi_{Omax} - 1]_{\mathbb{Z}}$. When the signal *cen* is low, the output register (and the complete incrementor-based counter) is cleared using the multiplexer controlled by *cen* (Figure 5.13).

Second delay line DL_2 is used to compensate the delay of the environment WCOEenv. The output from the delay line, signal *we_wc*, is the "data valid" signal for the weighting coefficient values.

Third delay line DL_3 is used to compensate the pipelining delay of the INSenv. The output signal we_ins is the "data valid" signal for the intersect values from the INSenv.

Algorithm 15 specifies the AGenv. Environment AGenv starts after activation of the signal st. The computations are performed from the center ($r_O = 0$) of the upper plane $z_O = 0$. These computations are done for all voxels on one radial element (z_O, r_O) only. This is the inner loop in the computation of the Geometry Table (Algorithm 4). The loops for the radial elements and planes are done by the environments of the Control Unit: PECenv (Algorithm 13) and CCenv (Algorithm 11) respectively.

First, the signal wen is activated. This signal stays active for ϕ_{Omax} cycles (lines 2-4) when the values of the counter ϕ_O are generated. After ϕ_{Omax} many values are generated, environment AGenv waits until the geometry computations are done, i.e. when the signal we_ins is low (line 6). Next, the value of the counter r_O is incremented and the environment AGenv waits for the next activation of the signal st. When the geometry data for all radial elements in one plane are computed, the plane counter is incremented (line 10). After z_{Omax} planes are processed, the counters of the AGenv are initialized to start the computations from the upper plane.

The control signal wen and the counters (in AGenv) are cleared on reset.

1: **if** $rst = 1$ **then**
2: $\quad \phi_O \leftarrow 0, r_O \leftarrow 0, z_O \leftarrow 0, wen \leftarrow 0$
3: **end if**

5.6.5 TSCenv Environment

The values of the transcendental functions are provided by the environment TSCenv. These values are stored in read-only memories (ROMs). The signs are computed in parallel with the access to these memories. The exploitation of symmetries of the

---
Algorithm 15 AGenv Algorithm

Require: signal st was issued in the previous cycle

1: $wen^t \leftarrow 1$

2: **while** $\phi_O \leq \phi_{Omax}$ **do**   *(generate counter ϕ_O)*

3:      $\phi_O^t \leftarrow \phi_O^{t-1} + 1$

4: **end while**

5: $wen^t \leftarrow 0$

6: **waitfor** $wi = 0$ *(wait for the end of the computations)*

7: $r_O^t \leftarrow r_O^{t-1} + 1$ *(next radial element)*

8: **if** $r_O = r_{Omax}$ **then**

9:      $r_O^t \leftarrow 0$ *(start from the center of the plane)*

10:      $z_O^t \leftarrow z_O^{t-1} + 1$ *(next plane)*

11:      **if** $z_O = z_{Omax}$ **then**

12:          $z_O^t \leftarrow 0$ *(initialize for the upper plane)*

13:      **end if**

14: **end if**
---

transcendental functions are not used, because this requires more complex control logic for the current environment.

The input of the TSCenv consists of two busses $\phi_O[\phi_w - 1 : 0]$ and $\phi_S[\phi_w - 1 : 0]$. The address values for the access to ROMs are transferred using these busses. The output of the environment TSCenv consists of the following busses and signals:

- the busses *cost* and *sint* are used to transfer the unsigned values of the cos() and sin() functions accordingly;

- the signals *cneg* and *sneg* are the sign signals for the corresponding values of the cos() and sin() functions.

The structure of the environment TSCenv is depicted on Figure 5.14. It consists of two ROMs with the values of the tables *sint* and *cost*, and the logic for the computation of signs (5.6.5). The value of the counter ϕ_O is used as an address for the memory *cost* and is an input of the comparators. The value of the cos() function and it's sign are ready at the output at the same time (the bus *cost* and the signal *cneg* respectively).

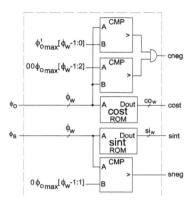

Figure 5.14: TSCenv Environment. By ϕ' we denote the constant value $0.75 \cdot \phi_{Omax}$.

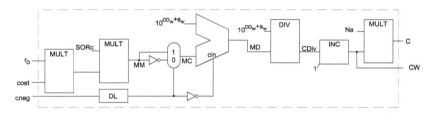

Figure 5.15: Circuitry of the COMTenv.

The memory with the *sint* values is accessed using the addresses from the bus ϕ_S. The same values from the bus ϕ_S are used to compute sign of the sin() function. Both, the values of the sin() function and the signs are ready simultaneously at the outputs *sint* and *sneg*.

5.6.6 Computation of the "Common Term"

Environment COMTenv provides the computation of the "common term" (Figure 5.15). This environment is an implementation of the Equation (5.6.1).

Two constants, Na and $SORc$, are used to obtain the output values

$$CW := \frac{1}{1 - SORc \cdot r_O \cdot \cos(\phi_{Oa})}$$

141

and

$$C := CW \cdot Na = \frac{Na}{1 - SORc \cdot r_O \cdot \cos(\phi_{Oa})}.$$

The computation of both values is performed sequentially in a pipelined structure: for a fixed value of the counter r_O in each cycle the new value $cost$ and the sign $cneg$ are received from the TSCenv.

The result of the multiplication

$$MM = SORc \cdot r_O \cdot cost(\phi_O) \equiv SORc \cdot r_O \cdot |\cos(\phi_{Oa})|$$

is an unsigned fixed-point number

$$\langle MM[r_w + co_w + s_w : 0] \rangle \cdot 2^{-co_w - s_w}.$$

Because the cosine value can be negative ($cneg = 1$), it goes through the multiplexer that is controlled by the $cneg$ signal

$$\langle MC[r_w + co_w + s_w : 0] \rangle = \begin{cases} \langle MM \rangle & \text{if } cneg = 1 \\ \langle \overline{MM} \rangle + 1 \pmod{2^{r_w + co_w + s_w + 1}} & \text{if } cneg = 0 \end{cases}.$$

We invert the value MM when $\cos()$ function is positive, because of the substraction in the divisor of the "common term". To compensate the delay of two multiplications, the signal $cneg$ is delayed by the delay line DL (shift register).

Before the division, we add the constant value to the MC

$$\langle MD[r_w + co_w + s_w : 0] \rangle = \langle MC[r_w + co_w + s_w : 0] \rangle + 2^{co_w + s_w}.$$

This corresponds to the addition of 1 to a fixed-point number with a $(co_w + s_w)$-bit fractional part.

The computation of the CW (5.6.6) is done using a divider. We divide a constant by the fixed-point number

$$\langle MD[r_w + co_w + s_w : 0] \rangle \cdot 2^{-co_w - s_w}.$$

Taking into account the fractional part of the divisor, the constant dividend is

$$\langle 10^{co_w + s_w} \rangle.$$

142

The output of the divider $CDiv[rem_w + 1 : 0]\rangle \cdot 2^{-rem_w - 1}$ is rounded using an incrementor - we add one to the lowest bit[11], i.e. performing "round nearest up".

$$\langle CDiv[rem_w + 1 : 0]\rangle + 1 \quad (\text{mod } 2^{rem_w + 2})$$

The value $\langle CW[rem_w : 0]\rangle \cdot 2^{-rem_w}$ is obtained taking $(rem_w + 1)$ leading bits after the incrementor.

The "common term" value $\langle C[rem_w + na_w : 0]\rangle \cdot 2^{-rem_w - na_w}$ is computed multiplying the constant Na with the value CW. This is a $(rem_w + na_w + 1)$-bit wide value, because $C \cdot Na < 2$ (we ignore the unused leading bit of the multiplication result).

The multipliers and the divider are the optimized pipelined IP Cores provided by Xilinx [82, 93]. We apply them (instead of "hand-written" modules) in our design only for efficiency reasons.

5.6.7   WCOEenv Environment

The environment WCOEenv is presented on Figure 5.16. It performs the calculation of the output weighting coefficient value $wcoe$ by raising the input value CW to the second power, and rounding this value using an incrementor.

The variable $\langle CWT[2rem_w + 1 : 0]\rangle \cdot 2^{-2rem_w}$ contains the result of the multiplication

$$\langle CWT[2rem_w + 1 : 0]\rangle = \langle CW[rem_w : 0]\rangle \cdot \langle CW[rem_w : 0]\rangle.$$

We perform the "round nearest up"

$$\langle T[wco_w + 1 : 0]\rangle = \langle CWT[2rem_w : 2remw - wco_w - 1]\rangle + 1 \quad (\text{mod } 2^{wco_w + 2})$$

and ignore the highest bit of the CWT because the weighting coefficients belong to the interval $(0, 2)$ (see section 5.6.2). The value of the weighting coefficient is obtained truncating the last bit of the variable T

$$\langle wcoe[wco_w : 0]\rangle = \langle T[wco_w + 1 : 1]\rangle.$$

---

[11]In literature this rounding technique is called also an "injection based rounding". For details refer to [92].

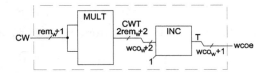

Figure 5.16: WCOEenv Environment.

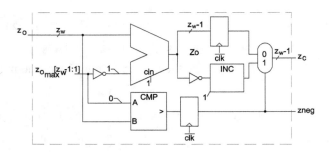

Figure 5.17: ZCenv Environment.

5.6.8 ZCenv Environment

The environment ZCenv is used to compute the the index of the current plane

$$z_c := z_O - \lfloor z_{Omax}/2 \rfloor,$$

which is aligned relative to the center of the volume. The structure of the environment ZCenv is depicted on Figure 5.17.

The signal *zneg* is used to indicate the sign of the z_c. It is defined as

$$zneg = \begin{cases} 0 & \text{if } z_O \geq z_{Omax}/2 \\ 1 & \text{if } z_O < z_{Omax}/2. \end{cases}$$

The signal *zneg* is an output of the comparator.

The value z_c is computed as follows. We compute first the offset of the plane from the center plane

$$\langle Zo[z_w - 2 : 0] \rangle = \langle z_O[z_w - 1 : 0] \rangle + \langle 1\overline{z_{Omax}[z_w - 1 : 1]} \rangle + 1 \pmod{2^{z_w-1}}.$$

144

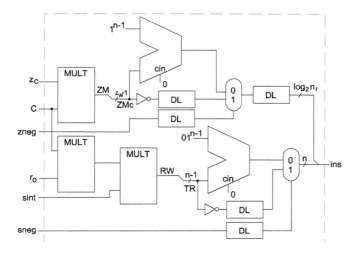

Figure 5.18: INSenv Environment.

After this, we invert the value Zo if $zneg = 1$ and obtain the absolute value of z_c

$$\langle z_c[z_w - 2:0]\rangle = \begin{cases} \langle Zo[z_w - 2:0]\rangle & \text{if zneg=0} \\ \overline{\langle Zo[z_w - 2:0]\rangle} + 1 \pmod{2^{z_w - 1}} & \text{if zneg=1} \end{cases}.$$

5.6.9 Intersect Values Computation

The environment INSenv computes the intersection addresses for the voxels of the radial element. The internal structure of this environment is presented on Figure 5.18. It consists of two parts that perform the computations of the vertical and the horizontal intersection coordinates. These two values combine at the output the intersection address.

Vertical Intersection Coordinate

This part of the environment is the implementation of the Equation (5.6.3). The coordinate z_d is computed using a multiplier, an incrementor and an adder. For the implementation we use $z_w = n$. This equality arises because the maximal number of planes z_{Omax} is comparable to the number of detector rows N (see (3.1.15) in

145

section 3.1.7), and $n = \lceil \log_2(N) \rceil = \lceil \log_2(z_{Omax}) \rceil = z_w$.

The absolute value of product $z_c \cdot C$ is a fixed-point number

$$\langle ZM[z_w + rem_w + na_w - 1 : 0] \rangle \cdot 2^{-rem_w - na_w}$$

which is computed as

$$\langle ZM[z_w + rem_w + na_w - 1 : 0] \rangle = \langle C[rem_w + na_w : 0] \rangle \cdot \langle z_c[z_w - 2 : 0] \rangle .$$

We take $z_w - 1$ leading bits of the result ZM and truncate other bits

$$\langle ZMc[z_w - 2 : 0] \rangle := \langle ZM[z_w + rem_w + na_w - 1 : z_w + rem_w + na_w - n + 1] \rangle .$$

The vertical intersection coordinate is obtained depending on the signal *zneg*, i.e. the sign of the index z_c.

$$z_d = N/2 - 1 + \begin{cases} |z_c \cdot C| & \text{if } zneg = 0 \\ -|z_c \cdot C| & \text{if } zneg = 1 \end{cases} \pmod{n_r}$$

We use that $N/2 \pmod{n_r} \equiv 0$ because both values (n_r and N) are powers of two. For the case $zneg = 1$ we have

$$\begin{aligned} \langle z_d \rangle &= \left(N/2 - 1 + (\langle \overline{ZMc[z_w - 2 : 0]} \rangle + 1) \right) \pmod{n_r} \\ &= \langle \overline{ZMc[z_w - 2 : 0]} \rangle \pmod{n_r}. \end{aligned}$$

Thus, the vertical intersection coordinate is computed as

$$\langle z_d \rangle = \begin{cases} (\langle ZMc[z_w - 2 : 0] \rangle + \langle 1^{n-1} \rangle) \pmod{n_r} & \text{if } zneg = 0 \\ \langle \overline{ZMc[z_w - 2 : 0]} \rangle \pmod{n_r} & \text{if } zneg = 1 \end{cases}.$$

If the value z_c is negative ($zneg = 1$), the plane z_O is projected into the upper part of the detector, i.e. if the plane is situated higher than the central plane we access detector rows with indices from 0 to $N/2 - 1$. If the plane is lower as the central plane (z_c is positive), we access another part of the detector. Thus, for the case $zneg = 0$ the addition of the constant value $N/2 - 1 \equiv \langle 1^{n-1} \rangle$ is required.

The value *zneg* is delayed using a shift register to compensate the delay of the multiplication $C \cdot z_c$ and the delay of the incrementor. The value $\langle z_d[\log_2 n_r - 1 : 0] \rangle$

146

is delayed after the adder in order to align it to the computation of the value $\langle ins[n-1:0]\rangle$.

$$ins[n+\log_2 n_r - 1 : n] = z_d[\log_2 n_r - 1 : 0]$$

Horizontal Intersection Coordinate

The horizonal intersection coordinate p_d is calculated using (5.6.2). The computation of p_d uses two multipliers, a multiplexer and an adder.

The absolute value of the variable RW is a fixed-point number

$$\langle RW[r_w + rem_w + na_w + si_w : 0]\rangle \cdot 2^{-rem_w - na_w - si_w}$$

computed using two multiplications

$$RW = r_O \cdot sint(\phi_O) \cdot C \equiv r_O \cdot |\sin(\phi_{Oa})| \cdot C.$$

We truncate the result of the multiplication RW and take $(n-1)$ bits. The leading bit of the RW is ignored, because the absolute value of $\sin()$ function is at most one.

$$\langle TR[n-2:0]\rangle := \langle RW[r_w + rem_w + na_w + si_w - 1 : r_w + rem_w + na_w + si_w - n + 1]\rangle$$

The value $TR \in [0 : N/2 - 1]_{\mathbb{Z}}$ is computed relative to the center of the detector row[12]. In order to obtain the component p_d of the intersection point, we have to add the constant value $N/2 - 1$.

$$p_d = N/2 - 1 + \begin{cases} r_O \cdot |sint(\phi_O)| \cdot C & \text{if } sneg = 0 \\ -r_O \cdot |sint(\phi_O)| \cdot C & \text{if } sneg = 1 \end{cases}$$

For the case $sneg = 0$ we have $\langle 0\,TR[n-2:0]\rangle + \langle 01^{n-1}\rangle$. For the case $sneg = 1$ we have to invert the value TR.

$$\begin{aligned}
((\langle 1\,\overline{TR[n-2:0]}\rangle + 1) + \langle 01^{n-1}\rangle \pmod{2^n} &= \\
\langle 1\,\overline{TR[n-2:0]}\rangle + \langle 10^{n-1}\rangle \pmod{2^n} &= \\
\langle 0\,\overline{TR[n-2:0]}\rangle
\end{aligned}$$

---

[12]i.e. relative to the central pixel with address $N/2 - 1$

Combining two cases, the output value $\langle ins[n-1:0]\rangle$ is computed as

$$\langle ins[n-1:0]\rangle = \begin{cases} \langle 0\,TR[n-2:0]\rangle + \langle 01^{n-1}\rangle & \text{if } sneg = 0 \\ \langle 0\,\overline{TR[n-2:0]}\rangle & \text{if } sneg = 1 \end{cases}.$$

5.7 Data Control Unit

The Data Control Unit together with the Parallel Backprojector is an implementation of the pipelined parallel backprojection of a radial element (section 4.3).

The Data Control Unit performs the scheduling of all processes, involved in the reconstruction of a radial element. It handles the geometry data, calculated by the Geometry Computation Unit, initiates the reconstruction of a radial element and controls the backprojection flow. The unit has an interface to the SDRAM chips that are placed in the external memory.

Interface

The input signals of the unit come from two modules of the design: from the Control Unit and from the Geometry Computation Unit. The signals, used to initialize the processes inside the Data Control Unit, are issued by the Control Unit:

- the signal $st.PE$ is a start signal for the backprojection of a radial element,

- the signal $st.wr$ is used to initiate the transfer of the filtered data in the external memory,

- the bus $Y[\log_2 n_r - 1:0]$ is the row address for the data transfer in the external memory.

The data from the Geometry Computation Unit are received using the inputs:

- the bus $ins[n + \log_2 n_r - 1:0]$ is an input of the elements of the Geometry Table,

- the signal we_ins is a "data valid" signal for the bus ins,

- the bus $wcoe[wco_w:0]$ is an input of the elements of the Weighting Coefficients Table,

- the signal we_wc is a "data valid" signal for the bus $wcoe$.

The design signal rst is used for the initialization of the unit.

The output of the unit consists of the following signals and busses:

- the bus $CA[a_w + 4 : 0]$ and the signal $CF.re$ are the outputs connected to the external memory system,

- the busses $A_{FMw}[\phi_w - 1 : 0]$ and $j_{FM}[\log_2 p - 1 : 0]$ are the address busses for the Parallel Backprojector,

- the signal $wrFM$ is a "data valid" signal for the data from the external memory,

- the signal $stADD$ is a "start" signal for the Parallel Backprojector,

- the bus $wcoef[wco_w : 0]$ consists of the weighting coefficient values, required for the reconstruction of a radial element,

- the output acknowledge signals $rdy.PE$ and $rdy.wr$ for the Control Unit.

Structure

The unit structure is depicted on Figure 5.19 and consists of several environments.

- The control environment DFCenv performs the generation of the control signals and the address values for the memory access.

- The environment GMenv stores the values of the geometry data received from the Geometry Computation Unit. It has two memory structures for the intersect addresses and for the weighting coefficients.

- The environment IFCenv is the interface to SDRAM chips. It supports the required operations to work with dynamic memory.

- The environment DSenv is used to delay the control signals. The delay is a compensation of the latency of the dynamic memory access, and the delay of the environments.

149

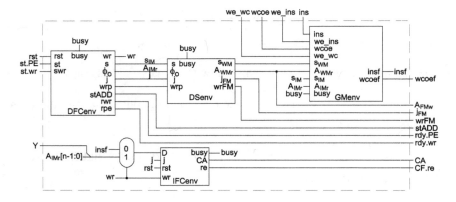

Figure 5.19: Structure of the Data Control Unit.

Computation Flow

Several different tasks are performed by the Data Control Unit: the access to the filtered projection data (read, write and refresh), the generation of the control signals for the Parallel Backprojector and the management of the input geometry data.

Depending on the input signals, one of two different operation modes of the Data Control Unit is selected: the "data transfer" or the "reconstruction" mode. The signal wr from the environment DFCenv is used to indicate the active mode.

- The "data transfer" mode ($wr = 1$) is activated when the input signal $st.wr$ is high. In this mode the transfer of the filtered data inside the external memory is performed (Algorithm 9 in section 4.5). Environment DFCenv starts to generate the values of the counters ϕ_O (for the elements) and j (for the rounds). These counters are available in the Data Control Unit on the busses A_{IMr} and j, accordingly. The values A_{IMr} are combined with the data from the input bus Y. The bus Y consists of the address value of the filtered detector row that must be transferred into SDRAMs. The SDRAM interface IFCenv receives the value after the multiplexer and issues the write commands (bus CA) to SDRAM chips in the external memory. The filtered data, that is written into SDRAMs, is fetched from the corresponding FIFOs (to these SDRAMs) under the con-

150

trol of the IFCenv. When the complete row is transferred ($p \cdot N$ elements in b external memory modules) the acknowledge signal *rdy.wr* is activated.

- The "reconstruction" mode ($wr = 0$) is activated by the input signal *st.PE*. In this mode the Data Control Unit performs the reconstruction of a radial element. The DFCenv generates the counters ϕ_O and j. The values ϕ_O on the bus A_{IMr} are used to read the intersect memory in the GMenv. The output intersect values are available on the bus *insf*. These values are used in the IFCenv as the address values for the external memory. If the row/bank change is required during the access to SDRAMs, the *busy* signal is issued by the IFCenv. This signal stops the update of the intermediate registers and the flow in the environment DFCenv. When the reconstruction of a radial element is done, the acknowledge signal *rdy.PE* is activated.

The value ϕ_O and the signal s (from the DFCenv) are used also to access the weighting coefficients memory (in GMenv). These values are delayed by the DSenv in order to compensate the latency of the SDRAM. The bus A_{WMr} and the signal s_{WM} from the DSenv are connected to the weighting coefficients memory structure in the GMenv. The output bus *wcoef* consists of the weighting coefficient values, that are aligned to the output values of the external memory. They are used further in the Parallel Backprojector.

The Data Control Unit generates the control signals for the Parallel Backprojector. These are the delayed counter of the elements (ϕ_O) and the counter of the rounds (j). The output signal *wrFM* is a "valid" signal for the data fetched from the external memory. This signal is generated only in the "reconstruction" mode.

In the "reconstruction" mode the DFCenv generates the signal *stA* at the end of each round j. This signal is delayed by the DSenv. The corresponding output signal *stADD* is a "start" signal for the Parallel Backprojector.

Environment GMenv receives and stores the geometry data, calculated by the Geometry Computation Unit. Using the corresponding "data valid" signals (*we_ins* and *we_wc*) the data from the busses *ins* and *wcoe* are stored in the RAMs of the

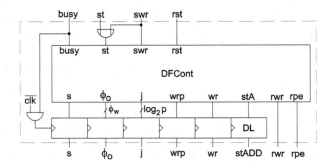

Figure 5.20: DFCenv environment.

GMenv. This process runs in parallel to the reconstruction of a radial element, i.e. in parallel with the access to the geometry data, stored during the reconstruction of the previous radial element. The GMenv has two memory environments: for the intersect data and for the weighting coefficients. These environments are the implementation of the doubled memory structure introduced in section 4.3.1.

5.7.1 DFCenv Environment

The environment DFCenv is a control environment in the Data Control Unit. It generates the counters and the control signals for other environments of the unit. The structure of the environment DFCenv is presented on Figure 5.20 and consists of the DFCont module and the set of the output registers. The interface of this environment is presented in Table 5.6.

Algorithm 16 presents the algorithm of the DFCenv. On reset ($rst = 1$) the signal s is initialized to 1 and the round counter j to 0. The signal s is set to 1 in order to select the memories in the GMenv, that will be filled with the geometry data for the first radial element before the start of the reconstruction of the upper plane (see Algorithm 7 in section 4.4).

The module DFCont of the environment DFCenv starts, when one of the interface signals is active.

$$DFCont.st := DFCenv.st \lor DFCenv.swr$$

Algorithm 16 DFCont Algorithm

Require: signal st was issued in the previous cycle

1: **if** $swr = 1$ **then**
2:     $wr \leftarrow 1$ *("data transfer" mode)*
3:     **while** $j \leq p - 1$ **do**
4:         **for** $\phi_O = 0$ to $N - 1$ **do**   *(elements of the detector row)*
5:             **waitfor** $busy = 1$ *(busy is active low)*
6:         **end for**
7:         $\phi_O^t \leftarrow 0,\ j^t \leftarrow j^{t-1} + 1$ *(next round)*
8:     **end while**
9:     $j^t \leftarrow 0,\ wr^t \leftarrow 0$ *(disable data transfer)*
10:    $rwr^{t+1} \leftarrow 0/1/0$ *(data transfer is done)*
11: **else**   *("reconstruction" mode)*
12:    $s^t \leftarrow \neg s^{t-1},\ wrp^{t+1} \leftarrow 1$ *("data valid" for the external memory)*
13:    **while** $j \leq p - 1$ **do**
14:        **for** $\phi_O = 0$ to $\phi_{Omax} - 1$ **do**   *(voxels of the radial element)*
15:            **waitfor** $busy = 1$
16:        **end for**
17:        $\phi_O^t \leftarrow 0,\ j^t \leftarrow j^{t-1} + 1,\ stA^{t+1} \leftarrow 0/1/0$ *(next round)*
18:    **end while**
19:    $wrp^t \leftarrow 0,\ j^t \leftarrow 0$
20:    $rpe^{t+1} \leftarrow 0/1/0$ *(reconstruction of the radial element is done)*
21: **end if**

Name	I/O	Width	Purpose
rst	I	1	reset signal
st	I	1	"start" DFCenv
swr	I	1	"start" data transfer
busy	I	1	wait signal of the SDRAM
ϕ_O	O	ϕ_w	address counter
j	O	$\log_2 p$	round number
s	O	1	select memory in GMenv
wr	O	1	"data transfer" mode
wrp	O	1	"data valid" for the external memory
stADD	O	1	"start" Parallel Backprojector
rwr	O	1	data transfer done
rpe	O	1	reconstruction of the radial element is done

Table 5.6: Interface of the DFCenv environment.

Depending on the input signal *swr* the environment DFCenv has one of two operating modes (they are operation modes of the Data Control Unit).

- *The "reconstruction" mode (swr = 0).* In this mode the DFCenv controls the reconstruction of a radial element. The address counter ϕ_O is generated from 0 to $\phi_{O max} - 1$ for p rounds, and $wr = 0$.

- *The "data transfer" mode (swr = 1).* In this mode the DFCenv controls the transfer of the filtered data in the external memory. The address counter ϕ_O is generated from 0 to $N - 1$ for p rounds, and $wr = 1$.

After start of the DFCont, the counter ϕ_O is generated in every cycle, when the signal *busy* is high, i.e. there are no wait cycles of SDRAM. If $busy = 0$, the value ϕ_O remains the same. This situation is expressed on the timing diagram of the "reconstruction" mode on Figure 5.21. For simplicity, by $INSM(A)$ we denote the value fetched from the intersect memory[13]. Assume that the values $INSM(A0)$ and $INSM(A1)$ are the addresses of the elements, placed on the same row and in the

---

[13]For the intersect memory see description of the GMenv in the next section. For the commands of the IFCenv refer to the description of the SDRAM interface in section 5.7.6.

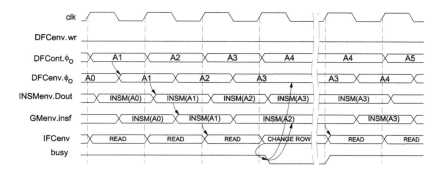

Figure 5.21: Timing diagram. Output address ϕ_O of the DFCenv is used to access the intersect memory INSMenv of the GMenv. The value $insf$ is received by the IFCenv and is decoded there. The *busy* is active low when the row of the SDRAM is changed by the IFCenv.

same bank in the SDRAM, but the element $INSM(A2)$ belongs to the different row. When the value $INSM(A2)$ is received by the IFCenv this environment activates *busy* (signal is active low), and the output registers of the DFCenv are stalled. The DFCont generates the next value ϕ_O and waits. After the row is changed, the IFCenv deactivates *busy* and the generation of the ϕ_O continues.

In the "reconstruction" mode, the DFCenv generates the "start" signal $stADD$ for the Parallel Backprojector. The signal stA is activated at the end of each round j. It is delayed by the delay line DL (shift register), which compensates the SDRAM latency and the delay of the environments GMenv and IFCenv.

The signal wrp is active in the "reconstruction" mode. It is a "valid" signal for the data, fetched from the external memory.

At the end of the process (the reconstruction of a radial element or the transfer of the filtered data), the corresponding acknowledge ("done") signal is activated: rpe for the "reconstruction" mode and rwr for the "data transfer" mode.

5.7.2 GMenv Environment

The geometry data, required for the reconstruction of the radial element is placed in the environment GMenv. This environment is depicted on Figure 5.22, and consists

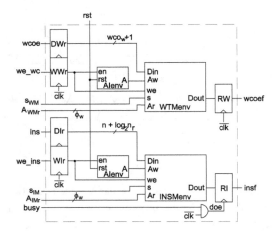

Figure 5.22: The structure of the environment GMenv.

of two equal structures for the intersect and weighting memory. Each structure includes:

- the input and output registers,

- the environment AIenv that is used for the generation of the write memory address values,

- the doubled memory environment for the geometry data.

The intersect addresses and the weighting coefficient values are stored in doubled memory structures (defined in section 4.3.1) - in INSMenv and in WTMenv, accordingly.

Interface

We divide the input of the GMenv into the several groups, as they are used inside the environment. The input of the intersect memory structure consists of the following signals and busses:

- the bus $ins[n + \log_2 n_r - 1 : 0]$ with the input intersect values and the corresponding "data valid" signal we_ins,

156

- the address bus $A_{IMr}[\phi_w - 1 : 0]$ for the access to the intersect data in the environment INSMenv,

- the signal s_{IM} is a memory select signal for the INSMenv.

The inputs of the structure WTMenv are similar to the inputs (of the INSMenv) described above: the input values are received using the bus $wcoe[wco_w : 0]$ and the "data valid" signal we_wc; the bus with the read address values is $A_{WMr}[\phi_w - 1 : 0]$ and the memory select signal is s_{WM}.

The common inputs are the rst used for the initialization, and the signal $busy$ used to control the output flow.

Data Flow

The geometry data is stored in the GMenv using the doubled memory structure (see description in the next section). The intersection addresses are stored in the INSMenv. The memories of the INSMenv store $(n + \log_2 n_r)$-bit elements. The weighting coefficients are stored in WTMenv. The width of these elements is $(wco_w + 1)$-bit. The signals s_{IM} and s_{WM} are used to select the memory inside the corresponding environments.

The reading from the INSMenv and WTMenv is performed using the values from the address busses A_{IMr} and A_{WMr} accordingly. The output values are available on the busses $insf$ and $wcoef$ through the corresponding output registers RI and RW. These registers are required to align the output data with the data flow in the Data Control Unit. If $busy = 0$, the register for the intersect data is not updated because it is clocked by the signal

$$doe := \overline{clk} \wedge busy .$$

This is done to stall the data flow in the "reconstruction" mode in the Data Control Unit. The output $wcoef$ is not stalled because the access to the weighting memory is performed using the delayed address counter (see description of the DSenv).

The INSMenv and WTMenv receive the values from the input busses ins and $wcoe$ through the registers DIr and DWr accordingly. These registers are clocked with the signal $\overline{clk}$ and pre-set the input data for the memories of the corresponding environments INSMenv and WTMenv. This is required because the memories in the INSMenv and WTMenv are clocked with the signal clk. The signals we_ins and we_wc are active when the data on the corresponding busses are valid. These signals are registered on input using two registers WIr and WWr. The outputs of the registers are connected to the inputs of the address generators AIenv. They are also the "write enable" signals for the corresponding environments. Consider, for example, the input signal we_ins. When this signal is active, the AIenv starts to generate the address counter for the INSMenv. The geometry data from the bus ins is written into the INSMenv using the write address on the bus Aw and the "write enable" signal from the register WIr.

The memories in the INSMenv and WTMenv are switched (signals s_{IM} and s_{WM}) at the beginning of the reconstruction of a radial element (signal s in the Algorithm 16). The Data Control Unit and the Geometry Computation Unit are started together by the PECenv of the Control Unit (section 5.3.3). The geometry data arrives with some delay after the start of the reconstruction because the Geometry Computation Unit is pipelined. Thus, the situation, that we write the geometry data twice into one memory of the GMenv, is eliminated. This means, that during the reconstruction of the radial element r_O the geometry data for the element $(r_O + 1)$ is written into the GMenv over the old data for the radial element $(r_O - 1)$.

5.7.3 Doubled Memory Structure

The doubled memory structure was presented in section 4.3.1 during the formal description of the backprojection. The circuitry of this structure is depicted on Figure 5.23. Two memories of this structure are denoted by the "RAM A" and "RAM B". Each memory stores $\phi_{O max}$ elements. The width of the elements is dependent on the application of this structure, e.g. for the intersect memory the elements are $(n + \log_2 n_r)$-bit wide.

The structure has the two input address busses: $Ar[\phi_w - 1 : 0]$ for the read address and $Aw[\phi_w - 1 : 0]$ for the write address. The input data bus Din is connected to

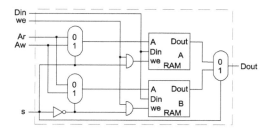

Figure 5.23: Doubled memory structure.

both memories. The input signal s controls the address multiplexers (here A_A and A_B denote the address inputs of the two RAMs)

$$A_A^{(s)} = \begin{cases} Ar & \text{if } s = 0 \\ Aw & \text{if } s = 1 \end{cases} \quad \text{and} \quad A_B^{(s)} = \begin{cases} Aw & \text{if } s = 0 \\ Ar & \text{if } s = 1 \end{cases},$$

the memory write enable signals

$$we_A^{(s)} := we \wedge s \quad \text{and} \quad we_B^{(s)} := we \wedge \bar{s}$$

and the output data multiplexer

$$Dout^{(s)} = \begin{cases} Dout_A & \text{if } s = 0 \\ Dout_B & \text{if } s = 1 \end{cases}.$$

5.7.4 AIenv Environment

For the simplification of the DFCenv, the generation of the write addresses $Aw[\phi_w - 1 : 0]$ for the INSMenv and WTMenv is separated into the single environment AIenv. The structure of the AIenv is depicted on Figure 5.24.

This environment generates address values under the control of the "enable" signal en. This signal enters the carry input of the incrementor. The data, that is incremented in every cycle, comes from the OAr register. The AIenv generates ϕ_O values from 0 to $\phi_{Omax} - 1$. The comparator signals the situation that the address value is equal to the design constant $\phi_{Omax} - 1$. When the output of the comparator is active, the register OAr is cleared. This register is initialized to zero on reset.

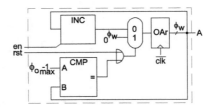

Figure 5.24: Circuitry of the environment AIenv.

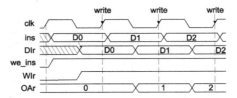

Figure 5.25: Timing diagram. Writing the input intersect data into the memory of the environment INSMenv.

The output register OAr is clocked by the signal $\overline{clk}$. The timing diagram on Figure 5.25 presents an example of storing the input intersect data from the bus *ins*.

5.7.5 DSenv Environment

In order to compensate the delay introduced by SDRAMs, environment DSenv delays the input signals. The delayed signals are synchronous with the data, fetched from the external memory. They are used later in the Parallel Backprojector. The structure of the DSenv is presented on Figure 5.26. The delays are organized by shift registers.

The access to the weighting coefficients memory (WTMenv in the GMenv) is delayed for the time, required to access the filtered projection data placed in the SDRAMs of the external memory. This delay is done by holding the values on the input bus ϕ_O and the input signal s for the time, equal to the CAS latency. The corresponding outputs are the bus A_{WMr} and the signal s_{WM}. The update of the output registers is controlled by the *busy'*. This is the signal *busy* delayed for the

160

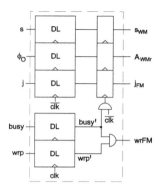

Figure 5.26: Circuitry of the environment DSenv.

time equal to the CAS latency.

The output signal $wrFM$ is a "data valid" signal. It is active when the data fetched from the external memory is available. The value of this signal is obtained as follows. The signal wrp is active in the "reconstruction" mode of the DFCenv. We delay the wrp for the time of the CAS latency in order to align the activation of this signal to the first element, fetched from the external memory. The output signal is active only at the moments, when the data from the SDRAM is available

$$wrFM := busy' \wedge wrp'.$$

5.7.6 SDRAM Interface

The SDRAM chips in the external memory modules are controlled by the IFCenv environment. This environment performs the following functions:

- initialization of SDRAM;

- read/write access to SDRAM chips;

- issue the signal $busy$ for the cases of opening/closing a row, a refresh;

- control the refresh of dynamic memory.

The interface of the IFCenv is presented in Table 5.7.

161

Name	I/O	Width	Purpose
rst	I	1	reset signal
wr	I	1	write access to SDRAM
j	I	$\log_2 p$	round number
D	I	$n + \log_2 n_r$	address of the detector element
CA	O	$5 + a_w$	SDRAM interface
re	O	1	"read enable" for FIFOs
busy	O	1	"busy" from SDRAM interface

Table 5.7: Interface of the IFCenv environment.

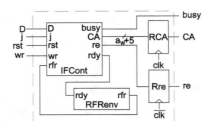

Figure 5.27: IFCenv environment.

The output bus $CA[a_w + 4 : 0]$ is connected to all b SDRAM chips, and includes the following signals: address $A[a_w - 1 : 0]$, RAS, CAS, BA, CS and WE. The control signals for the SDRAM chips (RAS, CAS, BA, CS, WE) and the control signals for the FIFO chips (WE, RE) are active low.

The structure of the IFCenv is presented on Figure 5.27. It consists of two environments:

- the environment IFCont that performs the control of the memory interface, and

- the environment RFRenv that controls the refresh of SDRAM.

5.7.7 IFCont Environment

The environment IFCont controls the dynamic memory interface. There are several variables and signals, that are used in the IFCont.

162

- A_R, A_{BA} and A_C are the variables, that contain the row, bank and column address, computed from the input busses D and j.

- The variables A_{curr} and A_{BAcurr} contain the address of the currently opened row and active bank in the SDRAM.

- The signal re is a FIFO "read enable". This signal is active when the data transfer process (SDRAM write) is performed.

On reset ($rst = 1$) these variables and signals are initialized. The SDRAMs must be powered up and initialized in the predefined manner with the following settings: CAS latency is set to 2, and sequential bank access mode is set[14]. This initialization is denoted by the ⟨ SDRAM init ⟩ in the description.

1: **if** $rst = 1$ **then**
2:    $busy \leftarrow 1, A_{curr} \leftarrow 0, A_{BAcurr} \leftarrow 0, re \leftarrow 1$
3:    ⟨ SDRAM init ⟩
4: **end if**

Algorithm 17 specifies the module IFCont. The process in the IFCont is performed in an infinite loop. The input data is decoded, and then the access to the SDRAM is performed. Depending on the currently opened row and active bank, this access can be made in this (the same) cycle, or the new row/bank must be opened (lines 3-5).

The input signal wr defines the type of the access to the SDRAM - read ($wr = 0$) or write ($wr = 1$). This corresponds to the operating modes of the Data Control Unit - the "reconstruction" mode, where we read the external memory, and the "data transfer" mode, where we write the new filtered row.

The address of the element (line 2), that must be accessed in the current cycle, is computed as follows (recall the description of the external memory structure from section 5.4):

1. The row address is $A_R^t \leftarrow \langle j\, D[n + \log_2 n_r - 1 : n] \rangle$.

---

[14]The init operation is not discussed here. For the detailed description refer to the datasheets of SDRAMs, e.g. [94].

Algorithm 17 IFCont Algorithm

1: **loop**
2:   ⟨ compute A_R, A_{BA} and A_C ⟩
3:   **if** $(A_R \neq A_{curr}) \vee (A_{BA} \neq A_{BAcurr})$ **then**
4:     $busy \leftarrow 0$, $re \leftarrow 1$, ⟨ change row and bank ⟩
5:   **end if**
6:   **if** $wr = 1$ **then**   (*check the operating mode*)
7:     ⟨ WRITE A_C ⟩, $re \leftarrow 0$, $busy \leftarrow 1$
8:   **else**
9:     ⟨ READ A_C ⟩, $re \leftarrow 1$, $busy \leftarrow 1$
10:   **end if**
11:   $A_{curr} \leftarrow A_R$, $A_{BAcurr} \leftarrow A_{BA}$
12:   **if** $rfr = 1$ **then**   (*check the signal for the autorefresh*)
13:     $re \leftarrow 1$, $busy \leftarrow 0$
14:     ⟨ Autorefresh ⟩
15:     $rdy \leftarrow 0/1/0$ (*acknowledge of the autorefresh*)
16:   **end if**
17: **end loop**

---

2. Assume that the filtered detector row with N elements is placed in the SDRAM row in two internal banks (as it depicted on Figure 5.8 in section 5.4.2). The memory row in each bank contains N/2 elements. Thus, the column address is $A_C^t \leftarrow D[n-2:0]$, and the address of the internal bank is $A_{BA}^t \leftarrow D[n-1]$.

When the currently active bank (A_{BAcurr}) or the opened row (A_{curr}) are not equal to those $(A_{BA}$ or $A_R)$, that must be accessed in this cycle (line 3), the active bank and opened row must be closed. This is done by issuing the following command sequence to the SDRAM

⟨ change row and bank ⟩ $\equiv$

1: NOP^t
2: PRE^{t+1} (*precharge the active bank*)
3: NOP^{t+2}
4: ACT^{t+3} (*open the new row A_R in the bank A_{BA}*)
5: NOP^{t+4}

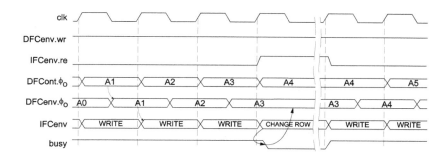

Figure 5.28: Timing diagram. The process of writing into SDRAM chips.

During this sequence the *busy* signal is low. This signal disables update of the output registers of the environments DFCenv and DSenv, i.e. the data flow in the Data Control Unit is stalled. In the next cycle ($t + 5$) the READ or WRITE command with the column address A_C is issued to the SDRAM chip depending on the signal *wr* (diagrams on Figures 5.21 and 5.28).

If the request of the refresh rfr is high, then the IFCont performs the Autorefresh of SDRAM chips (lines 12-16).

⟨ Autorefresh ⟩ ≡

1: NOP^t

2: PRE^{t+1} (*precharge the active bank*)

3: NOP^{t+2}

4: ARF^{t+3} (*issue Autorefresh command*)

5: NOP^{t+4}

6: ...

7: NOP^{t+k}

8: ACT^{t+k+1} (*open the row A_R in the bank A_{BA}*)

9: NOP^{t+k+2}

During this sequence, the active bank is precharged and the Autorefresh command is issued. After $(k-4)$ NOP cycles the bank is activated again. The number of NOP cycles is dependent on the SDRAM chip and the design parameters[15]. At the end of

---

[15]e.g. the time constraint of the SDRAM chip "Refresh to Activate" must be preserved [94]

the refresh the row A_R in the bank A_{BA} is opened again. The signal rdy is activated after the Autorefresh is ready.

If the Data Control Unit is idle, the IFCenv always accesses the element defined by the busses D and j, and refreshes the dynamic memory.

5.7.8 RFRenv Environment

The refresh of the dynamic memory is controlled by the RFRenv. Algorithm 18 describes the work of the RFRenv.

Algorithm 18 RFRenv Algorithm

1: **loop**
2:    $cnt \leftarrow 0$
3:    **while** $cnt < rfr_{max}$ **do**
4:       $cnt \leftarrow cnt + 1$
5:    **end while**
6:    $rfr \leftarrow 1$ *(request the refresh)*
7:    **waitfor** $rdy = 1$ *(wait for the environment IFCont)*
8:    $rfr \leftarrow 0$
9: **end loop**

The refresh control is done in the infinite loop. After rfr_{max} clock cycles the signal rfr is activated, signaling to the environment IFCont that the autorefresh of the memory must be performed. When the acknowledge signal (rdy) is received, the RFRenv starts to count the cycles again. The constant rfr_{max} must be selected less than the required number in the specification of SDRAM. This is done in order to control the situation when the signal rfr is activated, but the environment IFCont performs change of the row/bank and can not handle the autorefresh request.

5.7.9 Memory Access

The outputs from the IFCont, the signal re and the bus CA, are delayed using the registers Rre and RCA (see Figure 5.27).

The address and control signals of the SDRAM are delayed for one clock cycle for the reason that the data from the FIFOs must be available on the inputs of the

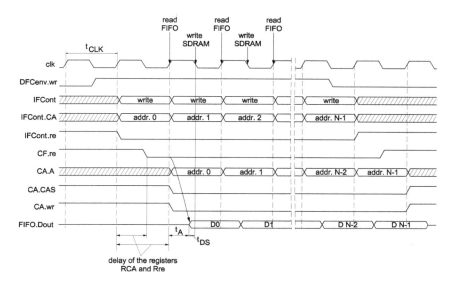

Figure 5.29: Timing diagram. Reading from FIFO and writing into SDRAM of the external memory.

SDRAMs before the writing[16]. This is described in the timing diagram on Figure 5.29. We consider one external memory module, and assume for simplicity (of the figure) that the write into the SDRAM is performed into the currently opened row and bank.

The data is fetched from the FIFO on the positive edge of the *clk* signal when $re = 0$ (the signal *re* is connected to the output *CF.re* of the Data Control Unit). The data is ready on the output bus *FIFO.Dout* along with the address and the control signals on the bus *CA*. The write into the SDRAM is performed on the falling edge of the *clk*. The parameters of the FIFO and SDRAM chips in the external memory are selected in such a way, that the "data access time" of the FIFO (t_A) and the "data-in-set-up time" of the SDRAM (t_{DS}) confirm to the following inequality

$$t_A + t_{DS} \leq t_{CLK}/2,$$

where t_{CLK} is a period of the clock signal (see Figure 5.29). This means, that data, fetched from the FIFO, must be ready at the input of the SDRAM in time less then

---
[16]This delay is counted by the delay lines of the DSenv in addition to the CAS latency.

167

the half of the clock period.

5.8 Parallel Backprojector

The Parallel Backprojector inputs the filtered projection data from the external memory, and performs the reconstruction of a radial element.

Interface

The following signals and busses combine the input of the Parallel Backprojector:

- the af_w-bit wide data busses $DE^{(0)}$ - $DE^{(b-1)}$ from the external memory,

- the initialization signal rst,

- the signal re_vm that is used to read the contents of the result FIFO,

- the busses and signals from the Data Control Unit:

  - the common bus $wcoef[wco_w : 0]$ with the weighting coefficients values,
  - the address busses $A_{FMw}[\phi_w - 1 : 0]$ and $j_{FM}[\log_2 p - 1 : 0]$ that provide the address values of the current element and the current reconstruction round,
  - the signal $wrFM$ that is the "data valid" signal for the data from the external memory.

The output of the Parallel Backprojector is the bus $VMout[res_w - 1 : 0]$ that is used to transfer the values of the reconstructed radial element. The output signal $drdy$ is a "ready" signal, issued when the result FIFO contains the backprojection result.

Structure

Figure 5.30 presents the top-level structure of the Parallel Backprojector. It consists of:

- the processing elements (PEs) that perform the weighting and storing the filtered projection data before the summation,

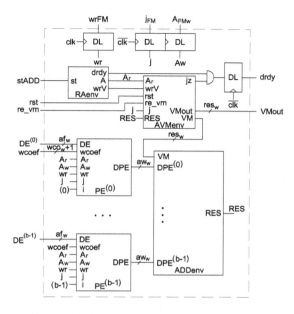

Figure 5.30: Structure of the Parallel Backprojector.

- the environment RAenv that generates the control signals for the environments of the Parallel Backprojector,

- the environment AVMenv that contains the volume memory and the result FIFO,

- the environment ADDenv that is a multi-port pipelined adder.

Computation Flow

The reconstruction of a radial element is started by the Data Control Unit (described in section 5.7) and is performed in p rounds (see formal description in section 4.3). The unit accesses the filtered projection data in the external memory, and provides the weighting coefficients and the control signals for the Parallel Backprojector.

The data, fetched from the external memory modules is received by the PEs on the busses $DE^{(*)}$. The number of the PEs is equal to the number of the external

169

memory modules. Using the weighting coefficients from the common bus $wcoef$, each PE weights the input filtered projection data, and stores the result in the intermediate memory. The writing addresses are computed by each PE from the value of the input address A_{FMw} and the values of the current round j_{FM} (reordering). The data is stored in the doubled memory structure.

At the same time, the data, that is weighted in the previous round, is accumulated using the adder in the ADDenv. The result of the previous accumulation round is summed with the new data and is stored in the volume memory of the environment AVMenv. The volume memory is a doubled memory structure. In the last accumulation round ($p - 1$) the data is written into the result FIFO. After p rounds, the result FIFO consists of the reconstructed radial element. The signal $drdy$ is issued when the last round of the accumulation for the radial element is started. This signal is generated by the RAenv and delayed to compensate the pipelining of the adder in the ADDenv. The contents of the result FIFO is read using the signal re_vm (see section 5.2.2).

The input signal $wrFM$ and the busses A_{FMw} and j_{FM} from the Data Control Unit are used to store the weighted values in the PEs. The data on these busses are synchronous with the input data from the external memory. The values on these busses and the signal $wrFM$ are delayed for the time, required for the multiplication of the input filtered data with the weighting coefficients in the PEs. The delay lines (DL) are organized by shift registers.

The read address A_r for the PEs is generated by the environment RAenv. This address is used also for the volume memory in the environment AVMenv to read the values of the accumulation result from the previous round. The RAenv generates the signal wrV that is a "write enable" signal for the new accumulated data on the bus RES.

5.8.1 Processing Elements

The reordering and storing of the input filtered data from the external memory is done by the PEs. The number of the PEs is equal to the number of SDRAMs in the external memory.

All PEs have equal structure and perform the same functions:

- compute the write address using the ordinal number of the PE,

- weight and store the data values from the external memory,

- provide the stored values for the accumulation in the pipelined adder.

Interface

The PE has the following inputs:

- the bus $DE[af_w - 1 : 0]$ from the SDRAM contains the filtered projection data,

- the bus $wcoef[wco_w : 0]$ consists of the values from the weighting coefficient memory (from the Data Control Unit),

- the address busses $A_r[\phi_w - 1 : 0]$ and $A_w[\phi_w - 1 : 0]$ contain the read and write address values for the weighted filtered data,

- the signal wr is a "data valid" signal for the bus DE,

- the bus $j[\log_2 p - 1 : 0]$ is used to transfer the value of the current round of the reconstruction,

- the bus $i[\lceil \log_2 b \rceil - 1 : 0]$ is a unique index of the PE.

The output of the processing element is a bus $DPE[aw_w - 1 : 0]$ used to transfer data from the intermediate memory in the IFMenv to the environment ADDenv.

Structure

The structure of the PE is presented on Figure 5.31. The processing element consists of

- the environment AFenv that generates the write address,

- the multiplier used to weight the input filtered data with the weighting coefficients,

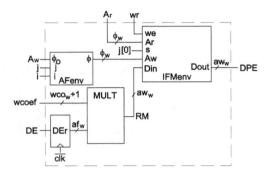

Figure 5.31: Processing Element.

- the environment IFMenv that is a doubled memory structure.

Data Flow

The input bus from SDRAM (that corresponds to the PE) is registered on the input of the FPGA (register DEr). The data from this bus is multiplied with the weighting coefficients values from the bus *wcoef*. The environment AFenv computes the writing address using the values A_w, j and the index i of the PE. The result of the multiplication is written into the environment IFCenv. This environment is an implementation of the memory $IFM_C^{(i,j)}$ from section 4.3.1. We used the doubled memory structure described in section 5.7.3. The memories are clocked with the signal $\overline{clk}$, and are selected by the signal $j[0]$, i.e. we change the memory in the IFCenv every round (recall that p is a power of two).

The output result from the multiplier $RM[af_w + wco_w : 0]$ is truncated taking aw_w leading bits (recall that the weighting coefficient is a fixed point number that belong to the interval $(0, 2)$)

$$IFMenv.Din[aw_w - 1 : 0] = RM[af_w + wco_w : af_w + wco_w - aw_w + 1].$$

An example of the data flow is presented on Figure 5.32. We depicted the delays of the address value and the signal $wrFM$, that are provided by the delay lines in the Parallel Backprojector.

172

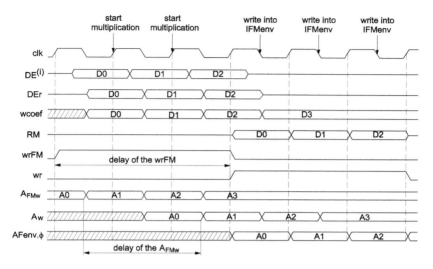

Figure 5.32: Timing diagram. Compute and write the weighted filtered data in the ith processing element. The pipelined multiplier has three internal stages.

AFenv Environment

Environment AFenv computes the address used to store the weighted filtered values. Figure 5.33 depicts the structure of the AFenv. The environment AFenv is an implementation of the formula for the reordering

$$\phi = (\phi_O - n_\phi \cdot (i \cdot p + j)) \pmod{\phi_{Omax}}.$$

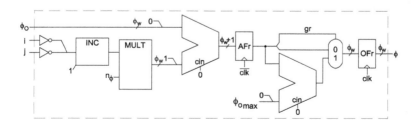

Figure 5.33: AFenv Environment.

First, the input of the multiplier is combined[17] from the input busses i and j as

$$(\langle \overline{i[\lceil \log_2 b \rceil - 1 : 0]} \, \overline{j[\log_2 p - 1 : 0]} \rangle + 1) \pmod{2^{\phi_w - 1}}.$$

The second operand n_ϕ is a design constant. Its value can be "two" or "three" (see description in section 3.1.1). In case of $n_\phi = 2$ no multiplier is required, and the result is simply the ϕ_w-bit number. For the timing diagram on Figure 5.32 we assumed that the multiplication $n_\phi \cdot (i \cdot p + j)$ is not performed because $n_\phi = 2$. For the case n_ϕ is not a power of two, additional cycles are required for the multiplication and they must be included into the delay lines of the Parallel Backprojector.

Second, the register AFr stores the result of the substraction

$$AFr := \phi_O - n_\phi \cdot (i \cdot p + j).$$

The $(\phi_w + 1)$-bit value in the register AFr is a two's complement number. The highest bit (the sign bit) $gr := AFr[\phi_w]$ controls the multiplexer. The value after the multiplexer is saved into the output register as

$$\langle OFr[\phi_w - 1 : 0] \rangle := \begin{cases} \langle AFr[\phi_w - 1 : 0] \rangle & \text{if } gr = 0 \\ (\langle AFr[\phi_w : 0] \rangle + \langle 0\phi_{Omax} \rangle) \pmod{2^{\phi_w}} & \text{if } gr = 1 \end{cases}.$$

5.8.2 ADDenv Environment

The environment ADDenv is used for the backprojection of the weighted filtered detector values, stored in the processing elements. The ADDenv consists of the pipelined adder that performs the summation of the values received from b PEs and from the volume memory (environment VMenv of the AVMenv). The result of the accumulation is send with the bus RES to the environment AVMenv of the Backprojector.

For the description of the multi-port adder we introduce the main elements of such adder, then describe the tree structure, and afterwards describe the adder of the ADDenv.

---

[17] recall that p is a power of two

Carry Save Adder (*k-3/2-adder*)

The main element of the accumulation structure is a *k-3/2-adder* described e.g. in the textbook [88]. This adder compresses the sum of the three *k*-bit numbers to two numbers, which have the same sum. These two output numbers is a carry save representation of the sum. The *k-3/2-adders* have the inputs $a[k-1:0]$, $b[k-1:0]$, $c[k-1:0]$ and outputs $s[k-1:0]$ and $t[k:0]$ satisfying

$$\langle a \rangle + \langle b \rangle + \langle c \rangle = \langle s \rangle + \langle t \rangle.$$

The *k-3/2-adder* is constructed from the row of full adders. The delay is independent of *k*.

From two *k-3/2-adders* we construct a *k-4/2-adder* [88]. This is a circuit with the inputs $a[k-1:0]$, $b[k-1:0]$, $c[k-1:0]$, $d[k-1:0]$ and outputs $s[k:0]$, $t[k:0]$ such that

$$\langle a \rangle + \langle b \rangle + \langle c \rangle + \langle d \rangle = \langle s \rangle + \langle t \rangle \pmod{2^{k+1}}.$$

Tree Structure

Let $h := b + 1$. We construct a $\mathcal{T}(h)$ addition tree placed in the ADDenv. The top level of this tree is constructed from the 4/2- and 3/2-adders. The number of these adders depends on *h*. The bottom of this tree structure is completely regular 4/2-tree. The output of the tree $\mathcal{T}(h)$ is a carry save representation of the sum of inputs. An ordinary full adder is used to produce the binary representation of a sum from the carry save representation.

For the upper part we use the *k-4/2* and *k-3/2-adders*. The number of these adders is obtained as follows [88]. Let M be a smallest power of two, such that $M \geq h$

$$M = 2^{\lceil \log_2 h \rceil}.$$

For the input of the tree we have to distinguish between two cases.

1. $3M/4 \leq h \leq M$. The number of the 4/2-*adders* is $a = h - 3M/4$, and the number of 3/2-*adders* is $l = M/4 - a$.

2. $M/2 \leq h < 3M/4$. The number of $3/2$-adders is $l = h - M/2$, and $h - 3l$ inputs are feed directly into the bottom tree.

The bottom of the tree $\mathcal{T}(h)$ is a $4/2$-tree $T(M/4)$. It has $M/2$ inputs and $M/8$ $4/2$-adders. The depth of this tree is $\mu_a = \log_2(M/2)$.

Multi-Port Adder

Figure 5.34 shows the structure of the ADDenv which is a tree $\mathcal{T}(h)$. Each stage of the tree has the intermediate registers: μ_a for the $4/2$-tree $T(M/4)$ and one stage for the result from the input adders. These $\mu_a + 1$ registers are clocked in the following way: first stage has clock signal clk, second - $\overline{clk}$, third clk etc. The register after the full adder is clocked with the signal clk even if the output register of the $T(M/4)$ is clocked with the signal clk. This is done in order to align the result on the bus RES with the input of the volume memory of the VMenv (in the environment AVMenv).

5.8.3 RAenv Environment

The address values, required to fetch the data from the PEs for the accumulation stage of the backprojection, are generated by the RAenv. This address is used also for the volume memory in the environment AVMenv in order to read the old and to store the new accumulated values for the reconstruction. The RAenv generates the "write enable" signal for the AVMenv.

The specification of the RAenv is given by Algorithm 19. After the signal st is activated, the RAenv starts the generation of the address values. The signal $drdy$ is activated for one clock period in order to signal the external device that the reconstructed data can be read from the result FIFO. It is activated on each start, but the output signal $drdy$ of the Parallel Backprojector is active only in round $j = 0$. During this process the output signal wrV is active, enabling write of the accumulated values in the environment ADDenv. After ϕ_{Omax} values were generated, the counter stops and the write signal wrV is deactivated.

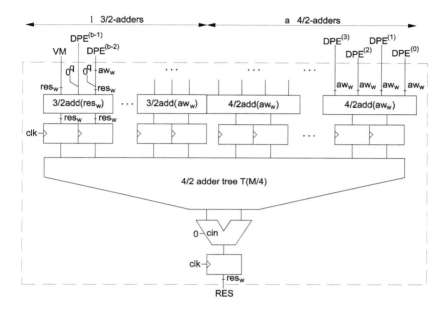

Figure 5.34: Circuitry of the pipelined adder in the ADDenv. By $3/2add(k)$ we denote the k-$3/2$-adder, by $4/2add(k)$ – the k-$4/2$-adder.

Algorithm 19 RAenv Algorithm

Require: signal st was issued in the previous cycle

1: $A^t \leftarrow 0$, $wrV^t \leftarrow 1$, $drdy^t \leftarrow 0/1/0$ (*write the reconstruction result*)

2: **while** $A < \phi_{Omax}$ **do**

3:     $A \leftarrow A + 1$ (*go through the radial element*)

4: **end while**

5: $wrV^t \leftarrow 0$

177

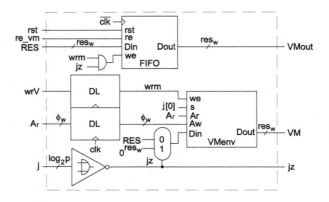

Figure 5.35: Structure of the environment AVMenv.

5.8.4 AVMenv Environment

The partial results of the backprojection of a radial element for $p - 1$ rounds are stored in the environment AVMenv. The result of the backprojection (last accumulation round) is stored in the FIFO in the AVMenv. The structure of the AVMenv is presented on Figure 5.35.

Interface

The input interface of the AVMenv consists of the following busses and signals:

- the initialization signal rst,

- the bus $j[\log_2 p - 1 : 0]$ defines the current round number and the bus $A_r[\phi_w - 1 : 0]$ has the address values for the volume memory,

- the bus $RES[res_w - 1 : 0]$ transfers the values from the ADDenv,

- the signal wrV controls the writing process of the values from the bus RES into the volume memory,

- the signal re_vm is a "read enable" for the result FIFO.

The output of the AVMenv has two busses:

- the bus $VM[res_w - 1 : 0]$ is used to transfer the values into the ADDenv,

- the bus $VMout[res_w - 1 : 0]$ is a output bus from the result FIFO,

and the signal jz which is active in the round $j = 0$.

Structure

The following elements are situated in the environment AVMenv:

- The environment VMenv is a doubled memory structure described in section 5.7.3. It stores the values of the accumulation. One memory provides
  the values for the accumulation, another is used to store the result of the current round from the bus RES. The VMenv is clocked with the signal $\overline{clk}$.

- The result FIFO is filled with the result values of the backprojection of the
  radial element. This is the memory VM_O from the description of the pipelined
  parallel backprojection (section 4.3).

- The delay lines for the address bus A_r and the signal wrV. These delay lines
  compensate the delay of the pipelined adder in the environment ADDenv.

- The zero tester for the input bus $j[\log_2 p - 1 : 0]$. The output signal from this
  tester enables write into the result FIFO.

Data Flow

The input address values on the bus A_{FMr} are used to fetch the contents of the
memory inside the VMenv and put it on the bus VM. The internal memory is
selected using the lowest bit of the bus j_{FM} and is switched at the beginning of each
reconstruction round j.

The values of the accumulation in the current round of the reconstruction are received by the VMenv from the bus RES. These values are stored in the environment
VMenv. Using the output of the zero tester

$$jz := \overline{\bigvee_{0 \leq k < \log_2 p} j[k]}$$

we control the accumulated data flow as follows:

1. The result FIFO is filled during the round $j = 0$. The "write enable" signal is computed as

$$FIFO.we := jz \wedge wrm.$$

2. During the round $j = 0$ the memory in the VMenv is cleared, i.e. it is filled with zeros for the reconstruction of the next radial element

$$VMenv.Din[res_w - 1 : 0] := \begin{cases} RES[res_w - 1 : 0] & \text{if } jz = 0 \\ \langle 0^{res_w} \rangle & \text{if } jz = 1 \end{cases}.$$

At the beginning of the reconstruction (the central radial element of the upper plane) in the first round $j = 0$ the environment RAenv is not active. Thus, the signal wrV is low and the FIFO is not filled. The FIFO is filled $z_{Omax} \cdot r_{Omax}$ times, because the RAenv is activated $z_{Omax} \cdot r_{Omax} \cdot p$ times. Hence, all radial elements go through this FIFO during the reconstruction. The contents of the result FIFO must be read by the external device using the signal re_vm (refer to Figure 5.3 in section 5.2.2).

5.9 Conclusion

This section presented the hardware implementation of the pipelined parallel reconstruction of the volume from cone-beam projections. The circuitry of the design performs all steps of the reconstruction algorithm: the filtering, the geometry computations and the reconstruction from the filtered projections. The described hardware design is implemented in the Xilinx FPGA with the external memory structure. The gate-level simulations provide the correctness of the proposed hardware architecture. The next chapter will discuss the results of the implementation.

Chapter 6

Evaluation

This chapter presents the quantitative analysis of the reconstruction hardware. We will describe the parameters of the design and their selection. We will discuss the characteristics of the design taking the parameters of the real application.

First, we describe the parameter space of our design. This will give the information about the practical problem and it's size. Second, we describe the simulations, that were carried out during the implementation of the design. Third, the preciseness of the geometry computations are discussed. We present the simulation results for the different bit-widths of the approximation coefficients. Fourth, the design performance and the parameters, that have influence on the performance, are discussed. We show the reconstruction results of the hardware Cylindrical Algorithm.

6.1 Parameter Space

The hardware design, described in previous chapter, was implemented in VHDL for Xilinx FPGA. Whenever it was possible, the design constants were changed into the implicit parameters.

The parameters of the hardware design fall into three major classes:

- Parameters of the tomography experiment. These values are used to determine the geometry of the reconstruction volume (see description in section 3.1). Table 6.1 contains these parameters with the example values from the real application. The size of the reconstruction volume, computed for the defined

Name	Constraint	Example
N	$N = 2^n,\, n \in \mathbb{Z}^+$	512
α	$\alpha \in [2.5°, 7.5°]$	7.5°
$\phi_{d\,max}$	$\phi_{d\,max} = p \cdot b,\, p = 2^k,\, p,b,k \in \mathbb{Z}^+$	384
d	$d \in \mathbb{R}^+$	0.4mm
m	$m \in \mathbb{R}^+$	2.0

Table 6.1: Parameters of the experiment.

experiment parameters, and some characteristic values are presented in Table 6.2.

- The approximation parameters are concerned with the size of the representation of the approximation coefficients, used for the geometry computations during the reconstruction (section 5.6.2). Bit-widths of these coefficients influence the size of the design and the precision of the geometry computations. The discussion about these parameters is presented in section 6.2.

- The scale parameters are concerned with the size of the design itself. They put the theoretical limit on the performance of the hardware, i.e. on the reconstruction speed. The parameters we consider belong to this class are the number of projection groups[1] b (recall the description from section 4.2.1) and the number of detector elements N (which also belongs to the first class of parameters). The widths of the data busses (Table 6.3) also belong to this class of parameters.

The values of the parameters, presented in this chapter, can be changed by a developer of the hardware system, for example, in case of changing the precision of the computations or increasing the speed of the system. The design issues, e.g. minimum clock time and the implementation specifics, are discussed in section 6.5.

---

[1] This is also the number of processing elements in the design that run in parallel.

Name	Value	Description	Section
z_{Omax}	448	number of planes in the volume	3.1.7
r_{Omax}	256	number of radial elements in one plane	3.1.7
ϕ_{Omax}	768	number of voxels in one radial element	3.1.7
L_{max}	59	maximal number of rows required for the reconstruction of one plane	4.5.1
n_r	64	number of rows for each projection stored in the external memory	4.5.1
TP	129	number of taps in the filtering kernel	5.5.2

Table 6.2: Parameters of the reconstruction volume for $N = 512$, $\phi_{dmax} = 384$ and $\alpha = 7.5°$.

Name	Bit-width	Format	Description
ad_w	14	unsigned	input projection data
fk_w	15	2's complement	filtering coefficients
af_w	32	2's complement	filtered projection data
aw_w	32	2's complement	weighted filtered projection data
rem_w	41	2's complement	reconstructed data

Table 6.3: Parameters of the data-paths of the design.

6.2   Geometry Computations

Here we will show the selection of the bit-widths of the approximation parameters used during the geometry computations.

6.2.1   Metrics and Parameters

We used C programs with floating-point and fixed-point computations (see description in section 6.6). The results of two programs were compared element-wise for the Geometry and Weighting Coefficients Tables. We used two metrics for the evaluation of the errors introduced by quantization (i.e. using fixed-point arithmetic) [19]. They are:

- Absolute error

$$\Delta x_i = |x_i^{\text{FP}} - x_i|, \ i \in [0 : M - 1]_{\mathbb{Z}},$$

where M is the total number of points, x_i^{FP} is the ith element computed using the floating point arithmetic, and x_i - using fixed-point.

- Average Absolute Error

$$\text{AAE}_x = \frac{1}{M} \sum_{i=0}^{M-1} \Delta x_i.$$

Table 6.4 presents the parameters (approximation coefficients) that were used in the geometry computations (section 5.6.2): the intersection coordinates (p_d and z_d) and the weighting coefficients ($wcoe$). The proper values, that are selected using simulation results are given in column "Bit-width". The selection of the approximation coefficients is discussed in the next section.

6.2.2   Selection of the Coefficients

Constraints

The following constraints were applied to the simulation results in order to select the proper parameters for the representation of the variables and constants for the geometry computations (section 5.6.2).

Name	p_d	z_d	wcoe	Bit-width	Description
co_w	+	+	+	7	cosine value
si_w	+	−	−	8	sine value
rem_w	+	+	+	9	remainder value
wco_w	−	−	+	7	weighting coefficient value
s_w	+	+	+	16	constant SORc
na_w	+	+	−	9	constant Na

Table 6.4: Computation values and the approximation parameters. Abbreviations: "+" parameter is used and "−" parameter is not used in the computation of p_d, z_d and wcoe respectively.

1. *The absolute error in the computation of the horizontal and the vertical intersection coordinates must be at most one* $(\Delta x \leq 1)$. This means that we bound the region around the correct intersection point. In case of the error computation (fault intersection value) the neighbor detector value will be selected.

2. *The error values on the bounds of the detector must be eliminated.* This is an extension of the first constraint and excludes situations, when the computation errors occur on the boundary values, i.e. for the pixels $p_d = 0$ and $p_d = N - 1$ for the horizontal coordinate, and for the rows $z_d = 0$ and $z_d = N - 1$ for the vertical coordinate. In these error situations the values are wrapped and instead of taking the neighbor value, the value with absolute error N is taken. We eliminate such situation by increasing the precision of the computations.

3. *The widths of the dividend, divisor and the remainder must be at most 32.* This is a constraint of the Pipelined Divider macro [95] from Xilinx Core Generator software.

Simulation Results

Extensive simulations were carried out in order to obtain the precision of the geometry computations and to select the values of the approximation parameters, that comply with three above defined constraints.

All simulations for geometry computations were done using C programs. These programs performed the calculation of the Geometry Table (see section 3.1.7) and the Weighting Coefficients Table (see section 3.1.8). We simulated the hardware geometry computations exactly as the computations flow in Geometry Computation Unit (using fixed-point arithmetic) for the following values: $s_w \in [11:20]_{\mathbb{Z}}$, $na_w \in [8:14]_{\mathbb{Z}}$, $rem_w \in [7:14]_{\mathbb{Z}}$, $co_w \in [6:14]_{\mathbb{Z}}$ and $si_w \in [5:14]_{\mathbb{Z}}$. The computation of the weighting coefficients were simulated[2] for the $wco_w \in [5:16]_{\mathbb{Z}}$. The simulations were carried out in the following way.

- The tables were computed using floating-point arithmetic (double precision). We assumed that these value were error-free.

- The intersect coordinates and weighting coefficients were computed for the five half-beam opening angles $\alpha \in \{2.5°, 3.75°, 5°, 6.25°, 7.5°\}$ for the fixed set of values s_w, na_w, rem_w, co_w and si_w from the mentioned intervals. These computations were carried out using fixed-point arithmetic.

- Each table (for each angle and for each set of values) was compared element-wise with the table computed using floating-point arithmetic. We analysed the errors for the horizontal and vertical coordinates separately.

The minimal values of the parameters, that satisfied the constraint $\Delta x \leq 1$, are presented in Table 6.4. We call these values of the approximation coefficients the *minimal values*. For the intersect coordinates we computed the average absolute errors: AAE_p for horizontal and AAE_z for vertical coordinate. These values are computed for each half-beam opening angle, and then averaged. The precision of the weighting coefficients computations was estimated using the values of the absolute error Δ_w.

In Table 6.5 we present results of the error estimation using two different sets of the approximation coefficients (from Table 6.4). The first set contains the *minimal values*. These values were used for the implementation of the design. One can see, that the precision of the geometry computation using these minimal parameters is low. In order to show the possible enhancement of the precision, we present the

---

[2]For the simulations of weighting coefficients computation other values of the approximation coefficients were fixed (we used the values that are presented in Table 6.4).

	Approximation	Error Estimation			Increase of the hardware	
	Coefficients	AAE_p	AAE_z	Δ_w	GCU	complete design
1	$s_w = 17$, $na_w = 11$, $co_w = 10$, $si_w = 10$, $rem_w = 11$, $wco_w = 7$	0.1384	0.0902	0.0073	–	–
2	$s_w = 20$, $na_w = 14$, $co_w = 14$, $si_w = 14$, $rem_w = 14$, $wco_w = 7$	0.0032	0.0041	0.0019	14.3%	1.2%

Table 6.5: Comparing characteristics of the design, using different values of the approximation coefficients. Abbreviation "GCU" is for Geometry Computation Unit.

estimation of the errors in the computations carried out using the maximal values of the approximation coefficients (second set). The precision is significantly improved using the bigger values of the approximation coefficients.

It was found, that the absolute errors of the weighting coefficients computations with $wco_w \in [5 : 7]_{\mathbb{Z}}$ are below the resolution of the corresponding fixed-point representation (numbers with wco_w-bit fractional part). Growth of the wco_w did not improve the accuracy of the computations. For the evaluation of the hardware we used value $wco_w = 7$ with the absolute error in the computations ≈ 0.0073. This error depends strongly on the parameters co_w and s_w, and on the value $SORc$ itself. This results in noisy reconstruction image, that requires post reconstruction filtering.

The errors in the geometry computations arise due to the quantization of constants (their fixed-point representation; see section 5.6.2). Also, the errors occur due to application of the standard IP Division Core from Xilinx [95], that has constraints for the widths of dividend and divisor (32-bit wide operands). In order to increase the precision of the computations, a special rounding for the divisor can be used. The computations can be performed with better precision ($co_w > 7$ and $s_w > 16$), and before the division operation the divisor has to be rounded to 32-bit value. This helps to compute the intersection coordinates and weighting coefficients more accurate. The side effect of this modification is that the hardware of the

Geometry Computation Unit (section 5.6) becomes more complex and size of the design grows. In Table 6.5 we present the estimation of this growth. The increase of the design size is computed relative to the size of the design with *minimal values* of the approximation coefficients. For the implementation we used the design with six processing elements. The evaluation of the design with better precision shows, that additional hardware in the Geometry Computation Unit does not increase significantly the size of the complete design.

6.3 Reconstruction of a Phantom

The spacial images, called phantoms, are generally used to test the reconstruction systems. One of the widely used phantoms is a Shepp-Logan 2D head phantom [43]. We used the equiangular projection data of this phantom from the open-source program CTSIM [44]. The projection data from this phantom was generated using the following parameters:

number of detector elements N	512
number of equiangular projections $\phi_{d\,max}$	384
focal length ratio	12.0
fan-beam angle	4.7802°
detector increment (d)	0.0103

We reconstructed these data as it were the projection of the central plane in the volume, i.e. the projection data were collected by a line detector with N elements.

The projection data was reconstructed using a C program. The program functionally simulates the hardware design: digital filtering, geometry computations using fixed-point arithmetic, integer backprojection etc. We applied the Shepp-Logan filter kernel (Equation (2.8.11)) with different number of taps. After the reconstruction, the data was converted to the Cartesian coordinates. This was done using the interpolation [66, 67].

Results of the reconstruction are presented on Figure 6.1. This figure shows the original rasterized phantom and the phantoms, reconstructed using different number of taps in the filtering kernel (see sections 2.8.2 and 5.5.2). Obviously, the quality of the reconstructed image grows with the increase of the number of taps TP.

The quality can be analyzed not only visually, comparing several images, but also using element-wise comparison. Figure 6.2 presents the density of the elements on the central column of the phantom[3] and the reconstructed image, respectively. The results are presented using the normalized density, which is suitable for visualization (grey scale). These figures show that the fixed-point reconstruction design can handle small (less that 1%) density changes. Figure 6.3 shows the reconstruction results using different number of taps for the digital filter (environment FLTenv section 5.5). One can see from Figure 6.1, that suitable results are produced starting from 129-tap filter, but this result requires an additional post-filtering after the reconstruction. The noise in the region around the phantom is produced by the filtering before the backprojection, and can be eliminated using the post-filtering[4] of the reconstructed image. This post reconstruction filtering is done to improve the quality of the reconstruction image further.

Further discussions about the improvement of the quality of the reconstruction result, e.g. using different filtering kernels are beyond the scope of this work because the selection of the filter is an application specific task.

6.4 Architecture Performance

The performance of the hardware reconstruction is analyzed describing the speed of the reconstruction and the bandwidth of the hardware architecture. Before this, the influence of the parameters of the reconstruction geometry on the performance is described.

---

[3]Comparison between the columns of the phantom and the same columns of the reconstructed image is a common technique, used to characterize the reconstruction algorithm.

[4]using the standard software, e.g. "VGStudio MAX" [96]

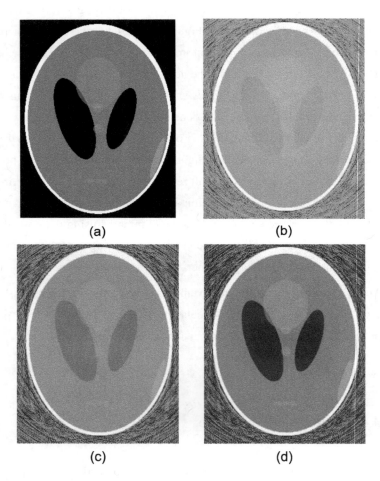

(a)

(b)

(c)

(d)

Figure 6.1: Reconstruction of the Shepp-Logan phantom. Figure (a) is a rasterized phantom. Figures (b), (c) and (d) are the reconstruction results using the 129, 257 and 513 taps filtering kernels, respectively. *All images are presented with the enhancement of contrast and brightness (for printing).*

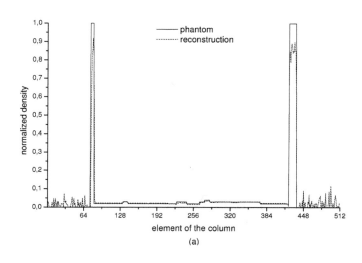

(a)

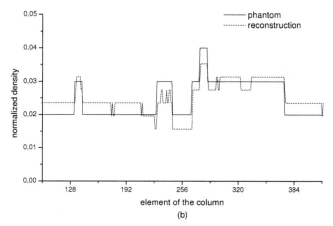

(b)

Figure 6.2: Central columns of the Shepp-Logan phantom and the reconstruction result with 513-taps filter. Figure (b) shows the central part of the column in another scale.

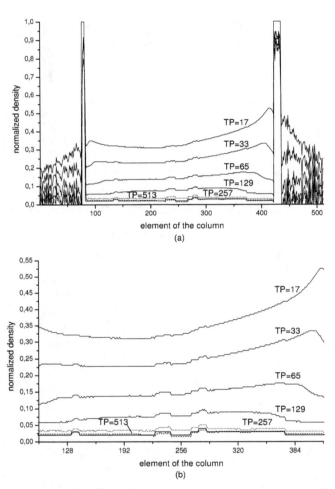

Figure 6.3: Central columns of the Shepp-Logan phantom and the reconstruction result using different number of taps in the implementation of the digital filter. Figure (b) shows the central part of the
column in another scale. Solid line on Figure (b) corresponds to the phantom.

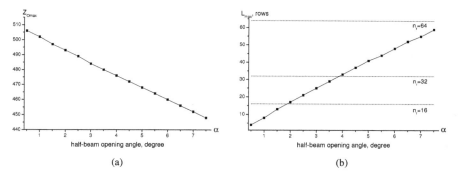

Figure 6.4: Reconstruction characteristics. (a) Maximum number of planes z_{Omax} in the volume. (b) Maximum number of detector rows, required for the reconstruction of one plane.

6.4.1 Volume Characteristics

The parameters of the experiment geometry define the size of the volume that is reconstructed from cone-beam projections (section 3.1). As an example we used $N = 512$ and $d = 0.4$mm. Two characteristics of the reconstruction volume (z_{Omax} and L_{max}) are presented on Figures 6.4(a) and (b). We describe the dependence of these parameters from the angle α. For description of α refer to section 3.1.4 and Figure 3.4.

- The half-beam opening angle influences the number of planes in the recon-struction volume (Figure 6.4(a)). The number of planes z_{Omax} is computed for each angle α using Equation (3.1.15).

- The plane, that situates on the top of the volume (and, symmetrically, on the bottom), has the biggest projection region, measured in the number of detector rows (section 4.5.1). For the Figure 6.4(b) we took data only for the upper plane. The projection region (number of rows) grows linearly with α. Max-imal number of the detector rows, required for the reconstruction of a plane, influences the size of the filtered projection memory (recall the parameter n_r from section 4.5.1). Thus, for the smaller angles α the reconstruction of one plane will be faster than for the bigger angles, because we access a smaller number of rows. In another words, the data is placed densely and we have to switch less rows in the SDRAM. This is discussed in the next section.

6.4.2 Reconstruction Speed

In order to determine the speed of the reconstruction of the whole volume we will start with describing the speed of the reconstruction of one plane. There are no additional operations between the reconstruction of two planes, thus we can generalize the reconstruction time for the whole volume using z_{Omax} and the speed of the reconstruction of a plane.

The reconstruction of a plane consists of two main steps: backprojection and filtering. As it was described in section 4.5.4 the filtering of one detector row is done during the backprojection of a plane. Thus, the time required for the reconstruction of one plane is combined from the time for the backprojection (section 4.4.2) and the time for the transfer of the filtered data into the external memory system (see section 4.5.3). It is expressed as

$$T_z = (N_{zbp} + N_{tr}) \cdot T_{CLK}, \qquad (6.4.1)$$

where T_{CLK} is a clock cycle time, N_{zbp} and N_{tr} are the number of cycles for the backprojection of one plane and for the transfer of the filtered detector row respectively. *Here we assume that only one detector row is filtered and transferred into external memory (see section 4.5.1).*

Backprojection

The number of cycles required for the backprojection of one plane is expressed as

$$N_{zbp} = \phi_{Omax} \cdot r_{Omax} \cdot p \cdot T_w,$$

where T_w is a coefficient, that considers the effects of using the dynamic memory in the design, and $p = \phi_{dmax}/b$. Recall that an access to a location in the dynamic memory requires several operations. If the accesses during the backprojection are performed to the non-neighbor locations, then the rows are often activated and deactivated randomly, and the hardware is stalled (signal *busy* in Data Control Unit,

194

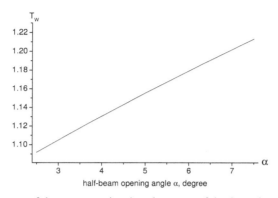

Figure 6.5: Increase of the reconstruction time due to use of the dynamic memory chips.

section 5.7). The number of detector rows, required for the reconstruction of one plane is defined by the position of this plane in the volume and by the half-beam opening angle (for example, see Figure 6.4(b) for the upper plane). The coefficient T_w includes these side effects. On Figure 6.5 we show the dependence of the T_w from the half-beam opening angle. For simplicity of the figure y-axis is the average value of T_w for all planes. Note, that T_w does not depend on the number of parallel processing elements, because SDRAMs work completely identical in parallel.

Transfer of the Filtered Data

The number of cycles required to transfer one filtered detector row (for all projections) in parallel from b FIFOs into SDRAMs is

$$N_{tr} = p \cdot (N + 10).$$

As one detector row with N elements occupies two rows in two internal banks of SDRAM (see section 5.4.2), we have to switch the rows during the data transfer, and to close the row after we have written one projection. This gives $(N + 10)$ cycles for each projection in total.

Characteristic	$b=1$	$b=6$	$b=12$	$b=24$
design size, Mgates	1.7	3	4.6	7.9
number of internal Block RAMs	23	42	66	114
number of inputs and outputs	152	314	511	907
design clock, ns	10	10.4	11	12.8
reconstruction of one plane T_z, s	0.87	0.151	0.08	0.046
reconstruction of the complete volume with $z_{Omax} = 490$, s	427.90	74.17	39.22	22.64
theoretical speed-up	1	5.93	11.71	22.79
simulated speed-up	1	5.77	10.91	18.75

Table 6.6: Evaluation of the design for different number of parallel processing elements b.

Initialization of the Reconstruction

When the reconstruction is started, $DLC[0]$ detector rows must be filtered before the backprojection of the first (upper) plane $z_O = 0$. The time for the filtering of $DLC[0]$ detector rows is expressed as

$$T_{init} \approx DLC[0] \cdot \left((N + TP + T_{wait}) \cdot \phi_{dmax} + N \cdot p \right) \cdot T_{CLK},$$

where T_{wait} is a number of clock cycles between the request of the detector data for filtering and arriving of data from the external device (sections 5.2.2 and 5.5.2). If the T_{wait} is a small value (see next section) and $DLC[0] \sim p$, then we can write $T_{init} \approx T_z/b$, i.e. the initialization is done faster than the reconstruction of one plane. The time T_{init} depends on the half-beam opening angle α: for the smaller angles we have smaller values of $DLC[0]$ (i.e. L_{max}).

Evaluation Results

Table 6.6 presents the results of the evaluation of the complete parameterized hardware architecture. We analyzed the parameters of the design for different number of processing elements b with identical parameters of the reconstruction geometry.

The speed-up of the design is obtained using theoretical and practical (simulation based) calculations. In order to compute the theoretical speed-up Amdahl's law was used [97]. It provides the limit of speed-up in terms of serial portion and parallelizable portion of an algorithm (implementation). According to Amdahl's law the speed-up $S()$ as a function of b is

$$S(b) = \frac{T_{zbp} + T_{tr}}{T_{tr} + T_{zbp}/b}. \tag{6.4.2}$$

Let f_s be fraction of our algorithm that is serial and cannot be parallelized. Obviously, this is a part of the reconstruction where the filtered data is transferred from $EIFM^{(i)}$ into $EFM^{(i)}$ in the external memory (Algorithm 9). We define this fraction as

$$f_s = \frac{T_{tr}}{T_z} = \frac{T_{tr}}{T_{zbp} + T_{tr}} = \frac{N + 10}{r_{Omax} \cdot \phi_{Omax} \cdot p \cdot T_w + N + 10}.$$

We modify (6.4.2) and rewrite it using the fraction f_s as follows.

$$
\begin{aligned}
S(b) &= \frac{T_{zbp} + T_{tr}}{T_{tr} + T_{zbp}/b} \\
&= \frac{b \cdot (T_{zbp} + T_{tr})}{b \cdot T_{tr} + T_{zbp}} \\
&= \frac{b \cdot (T_{zbp} + T_{tr})}{(b-1) \cdot T_{tr} + (T_{zbp} + T_{tr})} \\
&= \frac{b}{(b-1) \cdot \frac{T_{tr}}{T_{zbp}+T_{tr}} + \frac{T_{zbp}+T_{tr}}{T_{zbp}+T_{tr}}} \\
&= \frac{b}{(b-1) \cdot \frac{T_{tr}}{T_{zbp}+T_{tr}} + 1} \\
&= \frac{b}{(b-1) \cdot f_s + 1}.
\end{aligned}
$$

Results of the computations for different values of b are given in Table 6.6 in the characteristic "theoretical speed-up". Practical (simulation) speed-up is computed using values T_z relatively to the T_z for $b = 1$.

The efficiency of the hardware architecture decreases with growing b. The number of processing elements has a great impact on the size of the design and on the clock cycle time. When the size grows, the routing delays of the wires in the

FPGA start to play a significant role. Further discussion about the implementation in FPGA are presented in section 6.5.

The speed of the hardware reconstruction is significantly higher than the speed of a single PC reconstruction systems [6, 7]. The reconstruction time for a 512^3 volume from 400 projections is approximately five minutes. Running 24 processing elements our hardware architecture is faster by almost an order of a magnitude.

6.4.3 Bandwidth

Interface of the hardware architecture, described in section 5.2.2, has two important parameters: input bandwidth B_I and output bandwidth B_O. We will analyze the bandwidth for the case when only one detector row is filtered during the backprojection.

Input

The input of the design contains only the projection data from the external device. Recall the scheduling from section 4.5.4. One detector row for all projections (contains $N \cdot \phi_{dmax} \cdot ad_w$ bits) must be filtered during the time, required for the reconstruction of one plane, i.e. in $\phi_{Omax} \cdot r_{Omax} \cdot p \cdot T_w$ cycles. This constraint is required to perform the filtering of one detector row during the backprojection of one plane. Using that $r_{Omax} = N/2$ and $\phi_{dmax} = p \cdot b$ we obtain

$$
\begin{aligned}
B_I &= \frac{N \cdot \phi_{dmax} \cdot ad_w}{\phi_{Omax} \cdot r_{Omax} \cdot p \cdot T_w} \\
&= \frac{2 \cdot b \cdot ad_w}{\phi_{Omax} \cdot T_w} \text{ (bit/clock)}
\end{aligned}
\tag{6.4.3}
$$

On the other hand, the filtering of the complete detector row requires $N_{row} := (N + TP + T_{wait}) \cdot \phi_{dmax}$ cycles (see section 5.5.2). Recall that TP is a number of coefficients (or taps) in the filtering kernel, and T_{wait} is a number of cycles between the request of the projection data and the arrival of this data from the external device (see section 6.4.1). During this number of cycles (N_{row}) the $N \cdot \phi_{dmax} \cdot ad_w$ bits are

198

transferred into the design. In order to filter the complete row during the backprojection, the number of cycles for the filtering of a row N_{row} must be at most as for the backprojection:

$$(N + TP + T_{wait}) \cdot \phi_{dmax} \leq \phi_{Omax} \cdot r_{Omax} \cdot p \cdot T_w.$$

Thus, we can bound the number of cycles T_{wait} as

$$T_{wait} \leq \frac{\phi_{Omax} \cdot r_{Omax} \cdot T_w}{b} - N - TP. \qquad (6.4.4)$$

So, if the value T_{wait} confirms (6.4.4), one detector row can be filtered during the backprojection of a plane, and the input bandwidth is expressed by Equation (6.4.3).

Output

The reconstructed radial element (ϕ_{Omax} voxels) must be read from the design after the activation of the signal *drq* (section 5.2.2). This signal is activated periodically after $\phi_{Omax} \cdot p \cdot T_w$ cycles. For the complete plane we have r_{Omax} radial elements. Thus, the output bandwidth is obtained as follows

$$\begin{aligned} B_O &= \frac{\phi_{Omax} \cdot r_{Omax} \cdot res_w}{\phi_{Omax} \cdot r_{Omax} \cdot p \cdot T_w} \\ &= \frac{res_w}{p \cdot T_w} \text{ (bit/clock)}. \qquad (6.4.5) \end{aligned}$$

The values of the design bandwidth $B = B_I + B_O$ are computed for the different number of processing elements b, and are presented in Table 6.7. We used the parameters from section 6.1. The bandwidth results were computed for each $\alpha \in [2.5°, 7.5°]$ with step 1.25°. These results of the bandwidth (for each α) were obtained for the mean T_w for the whole volume. The values in Table 6.7 are the mean values for the bandwidth for different angles α. A standard interface controller, e.g. PCI of PCI-E bus controller for FPGA [98], can provide the required bandwidth for the hardware reconstruction system.

$b = 1$	$b = 6$	$b = 12$	$b = 24$
1.50	8.67	16.39	28.17

Table 6.7: Bandwidth of the design (in MByte/s) with the different number of processing elements.

6.4.4 Scalability

An important characteristic of the proposed and described hardware architecture is the ability to reconstruct the volumes with higher dimensions[5]. Usage of new detectors with $N = 1024$ or $N = 2048$ leads to enormous growth of the reconstruction time [6].

We have described our design as a parameterized hardware, thus simplifying the adaptation of this architecture for different sizes of the reconstruction problems. According to the analyses, change of the problem size, i.e. number of detector elements N and number of projections ϕ_{dmax}, leads to the linear change of the reconstruction time. This is due to the fact that the parameters of the cylindrical volume $(z_{Omax}, r_{Omax}, \phi_{Omax})$ are in linear dependence from the parameters N and ϕ_{dmax} (refer to section 3.1). For bigger N and ϕ_{dmax} our architecture requires a memory system with a larger capacity. Dynamic memories with capacities more than 64Mb are usually made with four internal banks with 256 elements each [94]. Thus, a slight modification of the hardware is required, because we provided description of the architecture with dynamic memory that has only two internal banks (for $N = 512$). In case of four banks, the coefficient T_w defined in section 6.4.2 will increase because the banks have to be switched more often during the backprojection.

For example, consider the problem with square detector $N = 1024$ and $\phi_{dmax} = 768$ cone-beam projections. The volume is eight times bigger than for our case with $N = 512$. Thus, the number of cycles for the backprojection of one plane will increase by more than eight times, and the volume will be reconstructed 16 times slower.

---

[5]By term "higher dimensions" we mean the larger sizes of the reconstruction problems, e.g. 1024^3 or 2048^3.

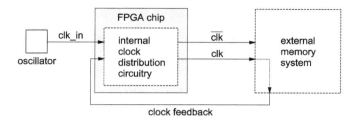

Figure 6.6: Synchronization in the hardware design.

6.5   Design Issues

Here we discuss the implementation of the design for the Xilinx FPGA.

- Design clock. The standard scheme using Digital Clock Managers (DCMs) [83] in Xilinx Virtex-II FPGA was applied for the clock distribution in the design. This scheme is identical to the example for the Virtex FPGA using Delay-Locked Loop (CLKDLL) described in [99]. We use two DCMs in order to provide the signals clk and $\overline{clk}$ for the design and for the external memory. This synchronization of the external devices (memory chips) is similar to [100]. Figure 6.6 depicts the synchronization scheme of the design, including the external devices. The signal $clkfb$ is a feedback for the first DCM. This signal is used for the compensation of the clock signal skew, introduced by the input and output pads of the FPGA chip, and by the trace of the clock signals outside the FPGA chip.

- All adders, accept the $3/2-$ and $4/2-$adders, are pipelined macros from the Xilinx Core Generator software [93].

- All multipliers are macros from the Xilinx Core Generator software. These macros use Virtex-II Multiplier blocks. We generated the macros using optimal packing option and with the maximal number of pipelined stages.

- All RAMS, ROMs and FIFOs are macros from the Xilinx Core Generator software. They use one-port BlockRAMs of the Xilinx Virtex-II FPGA [83].

201

- The environment FLTenv from section 5.5 is a Finite Impulse Response macro from the Xilinx Core Generator software. We used a 129-tap symmetric response filter with the constant signed coefficients.

- The algorithms, presented during the description of the hardware architecture (Chapter 5), are implemented directly as state machines using one-hot encoding [83].

The results of the implementation in the Xilinx FPGA are the following. We used Xilinx Virtex-II xc2v3000-6bf957 FPGA for the implementation of the design with $b = 12$ processing elements, and Xilinx Virtex-II xc2v4000-6ff1517 for the design with $b = 24$. The design was coded in VHDL with parameters, presented in section 6.1. The implementation was made using Xilinx ISE software [82]. Results of the implementation are presented in Table 6.6. We observe substantial increase of the design size using 12 and 24 processing elements. The size of the design influences the minimal clock cycle time T_{CLK} – it is significantly increased.

The components of the external memory, SDRAMs and FIFOs, are selected using the parameters N, n_r, p and af_w that define the capacity of the external memory system. For the values from section 6.1 we selected the following chips:

- b SDRAM chips from Micron [94] MT48LC2M32B2TG (2M × 32)

- b FIFO chips from IDT [101] 72V3xx0 (× 36).

These chips have compatible electrical standards of their interfaces, and can work on high (up to 133MHz) frequencies. Also, the constraint for the FIFO data access time (t_A) is preserved (section 5.7.9).

Here are some issues of the design implementation, used to increase the performance of our FPGA design.

- Usage of additional pipeline stages, that are not described in Chapter 5. These stages are required for better "place and route" technique [82], and they decrease the delays of the signals. For example, additional registers may be inserted before the first level of the pipelined adder array (environment ADDenv, section 5.8.2). This is done in order to register the outputs from the processing elements.

- Usage of divider implementation without the limits for the bit-widths of input and output operands. Solution is proposed in [102]. Increasing the precision of the division operation will impact on the size of the Geometry Computation Unit.

- The timing and area constraints were used during the implementation. The design was divided into time groups, and the specification of the signals from one group to others was made. This affects the run-time of the Xilinx software, but results in more optimal implementation of the design.

- Usage of a smaller number of taps in the digital filter (environment FLTenv, section 5.5.2). The number of taps strongly influences the size of the design, and the quality of the reconstruction result. The filter characteristics depend on the application of the design, i.e. what quality of the reconstruction must be obtained using the hardware systems.

- Usage of the newer software releases from Xilinx. The implementation of the design differs on the different software packages. As en example, we compiled this design using the previous software release. The performance was decreased up to 15-20% compared with result from the up to date ISE software. The newer software uses better algorithms and produces faster implementations.

6.6 Simulations

In order to analyze the characteristics of the design and to select the proper approximation coefficients for the geometry computations we performed different types of simulations.

Geometry Computations

- Programs in C language were written in order to obtain results for fixed-point geometry computations. These results were compared to the results of the same computations using floating-point arithmetic (see section 6.2).

- The approximation coefficients (their bit-widths) were selected by analyzing errors computed as the difference between the results of the fixed-point and floating-point implementations.

- The VHDL implementation of the Geometry Computation Unit was simulated in ModelSIM XE 5.2 (Starter version) simulator [86, 87]. The results of the hardware simulations were compared to the results of the fixed-point simulations programmed in C.

Backprojection

- The VHDL implementation of the Parallel Backprojector was simulated in the ModelSIM XE 5.2 (Starter version) simulator. The result of the backprojection (using arbitrary dataset) for one radial element was compared to the result from the C program (same dataset). They were identical. All functions in the Parallel Backprojector, for example, generation of the write addresses in the PEs, were tested using the C program.

Filtering

- A C program was written to analyze the different filtering kernels, that are applied during the reconstruction [54, 55]. Using the simulation results we selected the width of the filtering coefficients.

- The VHDL implementation of the Projection Filtering Unit was simulated in the ModelSIM XE 5.2 (Starter version) simulator, and the results were compared to the PC computations for the same data set (C program). They were identical.

6.7 Conclusion

In this chapter we have presented an overview of the hardware design implementation. The results of the implementation and the reconstruction examples were discussed. We analyzed the parameters, that influence the reconstruction time and the bandwidth of the hardware system. The time, required by the hardware architecture (with $b = 24$) for the reconstruction of a volume, is almost an order of the magnitude smaller than the time of a PC-based reconstruction system. We showed, that the speed-up of the system is almost linear with the number of parallel processing elements. A side effect of increasing the number of processing elements is the large size of the design.

We described the results of the simulations that were performed to obtain the preciseness of the fixed-point geometry computations. We analyzed the impact of the number of elements in the filtering kernel on the reconstruction quality.

Chapter 7

Summary

The problem of high-speed reconstruction is an actual problem for the 3D CT. Existing algorithms are under permanent optimization in order to increase the performance of the 3D reconstruction. Increasing of the detector data acquired for the reconstruction, for example, using newer detectors with the larger number of elements, can be handled only by applying the multi-computer systems. This is an actual and important problem in the field of NDT [6, 8, 60, 71]. If the reconstruction system has special size constraints (e.g. in industrial applications or in medicine), the use of currently available multi-PC systems is limited. Thus, the real applications force to investigate the alternatives for the large reconstruction multi-computer systems. These alternative systems must perform 3D reconstruction and have the performance comparable to the currently existing PC-based systems.

One of such hardware architectures for the reconstruction from cone-beam projections is presented in this work. The modified Feldkamp cone-beam backprojection algorithm (Cylindrical algorithm [61]) was implemented. In order to accelerate the reconstruction speed, first, the parallel processing technique was applied, and, second, the scheduling of the reconstruction was performed. All modifications of the original algorithm were formalized. Special analyses were made in order to define the minimal size of the memory, used during the reconstruction. The reconstruction is performed using fixed-point arithmetic. The flow of the fixed-point geometry computations was precisely described. The proposed architecture combines all steps of the reconstruction process: filtering and managing the projection data, computing geometry for the reconstruction on-line, and weighted backprojection of the filtered data.

The parameterized architecture was completely formally specified and implemented in Xilinx FPGA. The parameterized architecture was evaluated. Different characteristics of the implemented hardware architecture, e.g. size of the design, speed of the reconstruction, were presented. The impact of the parameters on the precision of the computations and on the speed of the reconstruction was analyzed. Additionally, the impact of using dynamic memory on the performance of the reconstruction was analyzed. Due to the formal specification and parameterized VHDL implementation the architecture is easy modifiable and scalable.

It was shown how the preciseness of the reconstruction is defined by the geometry computations and filtering. The results of the fixed-point geometry computations were compared to the results from the floating-point computations (C program). The constraints of the hardware computations were defined and the proper bit-widths of the approximations were selected. The errors of the geometry computations were estimated and their impact on the reconstruction was analyzed. It was shown that the relative errors of the on-line geometry computations are small - less than 0.001%. Thus, the impact of these errors is minimal. The biggest concern was the precision of division operation during the geometry computations – we used the IP Core Xilinx Divider v3.0. This Core has limitations of the input and output operands. One of the ways to overcome this limitation proposed in [102]. Using simulations, it was obtained that the filtering has significant influence on the reconstruction result. A Finite Impulse Response filter with a variable length filtering kernel was used. Obviously, filtering with low length kernel produces results, that require the post-filtering. However, the size of the filter has a great impact on the size and speed of the FPGA design [90].

The performance of the design was evaluated using a minimal clock cycle time of the implementation in Xilinx FPGA. One plane is reconstructed in time about 0.08 s[1], depending on the number of parallel processing elements, the position of

---

[1]for the 12 processing elements

the plane inside the volume and the experiment parameters. The 490×512^2 volume in cylindrical coordinates can be reconstructed[2] in 39.22 s using 12 processing elements and in 22.64 s using 24 processing elements. The time for the reconstruction of volumes with the higher number of voxels, e.g. 1024^3, can be computed using time required for the reconstruction of one plane (6.4.1) multiply the number of planes. These computations can be done after the evaluation of the modified design for the new problem. The clock cycle time of the design can be reduced using newer FPGA software, i.e. complete re-placing and re-routing of the design using new place and route algorithms. Nevertheless, the improvement of the design speed is almost unpredictable, because of the long routing delays of the interconnections in FPGA. We suppose that the result can be improved by about 10-15%.

The performance of the reconstruction hardware architecture was compared to a reconstruction system with Intel Pentium 4, 2 GHz processor. The time for the reconstruction of a 512^3 volume from 400 projections is approximately five minutes [6, 7]. The reconstruction of our hardware architecture is about an order of a magnitude faster for almost the same reconstruction problem. However, the technologies of the microprocessors and FPGAs can not be compared. An FPGA design has less functionality and is always slower because FPGA is a reprogrammable logic with long routing delays of the wires between the internal components. The memory technologies of the state-of-the-art PCs, e.g. DDR and DDR2, are also faster than SDRAM used in this architecture. Further increase of the performance of the hardware architecture can be achieved by:

- Using several FPGAs (several architectures running in parallel). This leads to a significant increase of the design size due to the large number of memory chips.

- Implementing the described architecture in a custom ASIC design. This helps to increase the design speed, which will be bounded now by the memory components of the design. The side effect of this solution is a high cost of the design.

---

[2] 512×512 plane square detector, 384 cone-beam projections

Bibliography

[1] S. R. Deans. *The Radon transform and some of its applications*. John Wiley and Sons, 1983.

[2] G. T. Herman. *Image reconstruction from projections - the fundamentals of computerized tomography*. Academic Press, New York, 1980.

[3] F. Natterer. *The Mathematics of Computerized Tomography*. John Wiley and Sons, 1986.

[4] A. K. Louis. *Inverse und schlecht gestellte Probleme*. Verlag B.G. Teubner Stuttgart, 1989.

[5] A. C. Kak and M. Slaney. *Principles of Computerized Tomographic Imaging*. IEEE Press, 1987.

[6] M. Maisl. Bauteilprüfung mittels 3D-Röntgen-Computertomographie. In *Blasformen '03, VDI-Gesellschaft Kunststofftechnik*, pages 183–193, 2003.

[7] SKYSCAN. Information available at http://www.skyscan.be.

[8] S. Gondrom, M. Maisl, S. Schröpfer, T. Wenzel, and M. Purschke. Fast industrial computed tomography and its applications. In *Proceedings of the 2nd World Congress on Industrial Process Tomography*, pages 265–271, 2001.

[9] D. A. Reimann, V. Chaudhary, M. J. Flynn, and I. K. Sethi. Parallel implementation of cone-beam tomography. In *International Conference on Parallel Processing*, pages 170–173, 1996.

[10] D. A. Reimann, V. Chaudhary, M. J. Flynn, and I. K. Sethi. Cone beam tomography using MPI on heterogeneous workstation clusters. In *Proceedings Second MPI Developer's Conference*, pages 142–148, 1996.

[11] F. Xu and K. Mueller. Accelerating popular tomographic reconstruction algorithms on commodity pc graphics hardware. *IEEE Transactions on nuclear science*, 52(3):654–663, 2005.

[12] D. Castaño Diez, H. Mueller, and A.S. Frangakis. Implementation and performance evaluation of reconstruction algorithms on graphics processors. *Journal of Structural Biology*, (157):288–295, 2007.

[13] Jr. E. E. Swartzlander and B. K. Gilbert. Arithmetic for ultra-high-speed tomography. *IEEE Transactions on Computers*, C-29(5):341–353, 1980.

[14] W. F. Jones, L. G. Byars, and M. E. Casey. Positron emission tomographic images and expectation maximization: a VLSI architecture for multiple iterations per second. *IEEE Tran. Nuc. Sci.*, 35(2):620–624, 1988.

[15] W. F. Jones, L. G. Byars, and M. E. Casey. Design of a super fast three-dimensional projection system for positron emission tomography. *IEEE Tran. Nuc. Sci.*, 37(2):800–804, 1990.

[16] E. Shieh, K. W. Current, P. J. Hurst, and I. Agi. High-speed computation of the radon transform and backprojection using an expandable multiprocessor architecture. *IEEE Transactions on Circuits and Systems for Video Technology*, 2(4):347–360, 1992.

[17] I. Agi, P. J. Hurst, K. W. Current, E. Shieh, S. Azevedo, and G. Ford. A VLSI architecture for high-speed image reconstruction: considerations for a fixed-point architecture. In *Proc. SPIE Vol. 1246, Parallel Architectures for Image Processing*, pages 11–24, 1990.

[18] I. Agi, P. J. Hurst, and K. W. Current. An expandable computed-tomography architecture for non-destructive inspection. In *Proc. SPIE Vol. 1824, Applica-*

tions of Signal and Image Processing in Explosives Detection Systems, pages 41–52, 1992.

[19] S. Coric, M. Leeser, E. Miller, and M. Trepanier. Parallel-beam backprojection: an FPGA implementation optimized for medical imaging. In *Tenth ACM International Symposium on Field Programmable Gate Arrays*, pages 217–226, Monterey, California, 2002.

[20] L. A. Feldkamp, L. C. Davis, and J. W. Kress. Practical cone-beam algorithm. *J. Opt. Soc. Amer.*, 1(A6):612–619, 1984.

[21] Cone-beam CT reconstruction server. Preprint, available at http://www.terarecon.com.

[22] M. Trepanier and I. Goddard. Adjunct processors in embedded medical imaging systems. In *Proc. SPIE vol. 4681, Medical Imaging: Visualization, Image-Guided Procedures and Display*, pages 416–424, 2002.

[23] Mercury Computer Systems, Inc. Information available at http://www.mc.com.

[24] P. Toft. *The Radon transform. Theory and implementation.* PhD thesis, Dep. of Math. Modelling, Technical University of Denmark, 1996.

[25] H. Hu. Multi-slice helical CT: Scan and reconstruction. *Medical Physics*, (26(1)):5–18, 1999.

[26] A. Poularikas. *The Transforms and Applications Handbook.* Boca Raton: CRC Press, 1996.

[27] H. K. Tuy. An inversion formula for cone-beam reconstruction. *SIAM J. Appl. Math.*, 43:546–552, 1983.

[28] H. H. Barrett and W. Swindell. *Radiologic Imaging.* Academic Press, New York, 1981.

[29] G. L. Zeng and G. T. Gullberg. Short-scan cone beam algorithm for circular and non-circular detector orbits. *SPIE Medical Imaging IV: Image Processing*, 1233:453–463, 1990.

[30] G. L. Zeng and G. T. Gullberg. Short-scan fan beam algorithm for non-circular detector orbits. *SPIE Image Processing*, 1445:332–340, 1991.

[31] F. Natterer. Numerical methods in tomography. *Acta Numerica*, pages 1–100, 1999.

[32] G. Wang, C. R. Crawford, and W. A. Kalender. Guest editorial: Multi-row-detector spiral/helical CT. *IEEE Trans. Med. Imag.*, 19:817–821, 2000.

[33] J. D. O'Sullivan. A fast sinc function gridding algorithm for Fourier inversion in computer tomography. *IEEE Trans. Med. Imag.*, MI-4(4):200–207, 1995.

[34] P. R. Edholm and G.T. Herman. Linograms in image reconstruction from projections. *IEEE Trans. Med. Imag. Vol.*, MI-6(4):301–307, 1987.

[35] J. I. Jackson, C. H. Meyer, D. G. Nishimura, and A. Macovski. Selection of a convolution function for Fourier inversion using gridding. *IEEE Trans. Med. Imag. Vol.*, MI-10(3):473–478, 1991.

[36] H. Schomberg and J. Timmer. The gridding method for image reconstruction by Fourier transform. *IEEE Trans. Med. Imag.*, 14:596–607, 1995.

[37] C. Jacobson. *Fourier methods in 3D-reconstructions from cone-beam data.* PhD thesis, Department of Electrical Engineering Linköpig University, 1996.

[38] A. Boag, Y. Bresler, and E. Michielssen. A multilevel domain decomposition algorithm for fast $O(n^2 \log_2 n)$ reprojection of tomographic images. *IEEE Trans. on Image Proc.*, 9:1573–1582, 2000.

[39] S. Basu and Y. Bresler. $O(n^2 \log_2 n)$ filtered backprojection reconstruction algorithm for tomography. *IEEE Trans. on Image Proc.*, 9:1760–1773, 2000.

[40] T. Rodet, P. Grangeat, and L. Desbat. Multifrequential algorithm for fast 3D reconstruction. *The Sixth International Meeting on Fully Three-Dimensional Image Reconstruction in Radiology and Nuclear Medicine*, 2001.

[41] H. Turbell. *Cone-beam reconstruction using Filtered Backprojection*. PhD thesis, Department of Electrical Engineering Linköpig University, 2001.

[42] S. Basu and Y. Bresler. Error analysis and performance optimization of fast hierarchical backprojection algorithms. *IEEE Trans. on Image Proc.*, 10:1103–1117, 2001.

[43] L. A. Shepp and B. F. Logan. The Fourier reconstruction of a head section. *IEEE Trans. Nucl. Sci.*, NS-21:21–43, 1974.

[44] K. M. Rosenberg. The Open Source Computed Tomography Simulator. Available at http://www.ctsim.org/.

[45] T. F. Budinger and G. T. Gullberg. Three-dimensional reconstruction in nuclear medicine emission imaging. *IEEE Trans. on Nucl. Sci.*, Ns-21:2–20, 1974.

[46] J. G. Colsher. Iterative three-dimensional image reconstruction from tomographic projections. *Computer Graphics and image processing*, (6):513–537, 1977.

[47] R. Gordon. A tutorial on ART. *IEEE Trans. on Nucl. Sci.*, NS-21:78–92, 1974.

[48] A. H. Andersen and A. C. Kak. Simultaneous algebraic reconstruction technique (SART): A superior implementation of the ART algorithm. *Ultrason. Imaging*, (6):81–94, 1984.

[49] P.-E. Danielsson. Iterative techniques for projection and backprojection. Technical Report LiTH-ISY-R-1960, Department of Electrical Engineering Linköpig University, 1997.

[50] K. Mueller. *Fast and accurate three-dimensional reconstruction from cone-beam projection data using algebraic methods*. PhD thesis, The Ohio State University, 1998.

[51] K. Mueller, R. Yagel, and J. J. Wheller. Fast implementations of algebraic methods for three-dimensional reconstruction from cone-beam data. *IEEE Trans. Med. Imag.*, 18(6):538–548, 1999.

[52] J. G. Webster. *Wiley Encyclopedia of electrical and electronics engineering*. John Wiley and Sons, 1999.

[53] G. N. Ramachandran and A. V. Lakshminarayanan. Three-dimensional reconstruction from radiographs and electron micrographs: application of convolutions instead of Fourier transforms. *Proc. Nat. Acad. Sci., USA*, 68(9):2236–2240, 1971.

[54] G. T. Herman and T. Chang. A scientific study of filter selection for a fan-beam convolution reconstruction algorithm. *SIAM J. Appl. Math.*, 39(1):83–105, 1980.

[55] S. K. Kenue and J. F. Greenleaf. Efficient convolution kernels for computerized tomography. *Ultrasonic Imaging*, (1):232–244, 1979.

[56] G. Wang, T.-H. Lin, P.-C. Cheng, and D. M. Shinozaki. A genaral cone-beam reconstruction algorithm. *IEEE Trans. Med. Imag.*, 12:486–496, 1993.

[57] G. Wang, S. Y. Zhao, and P.-C. Cheng. Exact and approximate cone-beam X-ray microtomography. *Focus on Multidimensional Microscopy*, 1:233–261, 1999.

[58] G. Wang, T. H. Lin, and P. C. Cheng. Error analysis on the generalized Feldkamp cone-beam algorithm. *Journal of Scanning Microscopy*, 17:361–370, 1995.

[59] M. Iacoboni, J.-C. Baron, R. S. J. Frackowiak, J. C. Mazziotta, and G. L. Lenzi. Emission tomography contribution to clinical neurology. *Clinical Neurophysiology*, 110:2–23, 1999.

[60] M. Kröning, T. Jentsch, M. Maisl, and H. Reiter. Non-destructive testing and process control using X-ray methods and radioisotopes. In *International Conference on Applications of Radioisotopes and Radiation in Industrial Development*, pages 21–34, Mumbai, India, 1998.

[61] Joachim Buck. *Schnelles Rekonstruktionsverfahren für die 3D-Röntgen-Computertomo-graphie in der Materialprüfung*. PhD thesis, Saarbrücken, Universität, 1996.

[62] Fraunhofer-Institut für zerstörungsfreie Prüfverfahren (IZFP). Information available at http://www.izfp.fraunhofer.de.

[63] J. Buck, M. Maisl, and M. Reiter. The cylinder algorithm - an efficient reconstruction algorithm for the 3D X-ray computed tomography (3D-CT) in NDT. In *Topical Conference on ASNT Industrial Computed Tomography*, pages 89–93, Huntsville, Alabama, 1996.

[64] A. Shih, G. Wang, and P. C. Cheng. A fast algorithm for X-ray cone-beam microtomography. *Microscopy and Microanalysis*, (7):13–23, 2001.

[65] G. F. Knoll. *Radiation detection and measurements*. John Wiley and Sons, 1979.

[66] N. Niki, T. Mizutani, and Y. Takahashi. A high-speed computerized tomography image reconstruction using direct two-dimensional Fourier Transform method. *Systems Computers Controls*, 14(3):56–65, 1983.

[67] H. Stark, J. W. Woods, I. Paul, and R. Hingorani. Direct Fourier reconstruction computer tomography. *IEEE Transactions on Acoustics, Speech, and Signal Processing*, ASSP-29:237–244, 1981.

[68] Z. Haque. *Investigation of computer structure for industrial computer tomography*. PhD thesis, Technical Universität, Vienna, 1991.

[69] M. L. Egger, A. H. Scheurer, C. Joseph, and C. Morel. High-performance scalable parallel platform for volume reconstruction of PET data. *Int. J. Imaging Syst. Technol.*, 9:455–462, 1998.

[70] W. L. Nowinski. Parallel implementation of the convolution method in image reconstruction. In *CONPAR 90 - VAPP IV, Joint International Conference on Vector and Parallel Processing*, pages 355–364, 1990.

[71] M. Maisl and S. Gondrom. Computerized tomography. *NDT in Progress*, pages 119–128, 2001.

[72] C. Laurent. *Adéquation algorithmes et architectures parallèles pour la reconstruction 3D en tomographie X*. PhD thesis, Université Claude Bernard LYON 1, 1996.

[73] St. Vollmar, C. Michel, J. T. Treffert, D. Newport, C. Knöss, K. Wienhard, and W.-D. Heiss. HeinzelCluster: Accelerated reconstruction for FORE and OSEM3D. *The Sixth International Meeting on Fully Three-Dimensional Image Reconstruction in Radiology and Nuclear Medicine*, 2001.

[74] C. M. Chen, S.-Y. Lee, and Z.H. Cho. A parallel implementation of 3-D CT image reconstruction on hypercube multiprocessor. *IEEE Trans. on Med. Imag.*, 37:1333–1346, 1990.

[75] C. M. Chen. An efficient four-connected parallel system for PET image reconstruction. *Parallel Computing*, 24:1499–1522, 1998.

[76] J. B. T. M. Roerdink and M. A. Westenberg. Data-parallel tomographic reconstruction: A comparison of filtered backprojection and direct Fourier reconstruction. *Parallel Computing*, 24:2129–2142, 1998.

[77] HAPEG Hattinger Prüf- und Entwicklungs- GmbH. Information available at http://www.hapeg.de.

[78] K. Rajan, L. M. Patnaik, and J. Ramakrishna. High-speed computation of the EM algorithm for PET image reconstruction. *IEEE Tran. Nuc. Sci.*, 41(5):1721–1728, 1994.

[79] K. Rajan, L. M. Patnaik, and J. Ramakrishna. High-speed parallel implementation of a modified PBR algorithm on DSP-based EH topology. *IEEE Tran. Nuc. Sci.*, 44(4):1658–1672, 1997.

[80] K. Rajan and L. M. Patnaik. CBP and ART image reconstruction algorithms on media and DSP processors. *Microprocessors and Microsystems*, 25:233–238, 2001.

[81] Frank Dachille IX. *Algorithms and Architectures for Realistic Volume Imaging*. PhD thesis, State University of New York, 2002.

[82] Xilinx Inc., Xilinx FPGA device manuals. Available at `http://www.xilinx.com`.

[83] Xilinx Inc. *Xilinx. Virtex-II Platform FPGA Handbook*, 2001.

[84] IEEE std. 1076-1987. IEEE standard VHDL reference manual, 1987.

[85] P. J. Ashenden. *The VHDL Cookbook. First edition*. Dept. Computer Science University of Adelaide South Australia, 1990.

[86] ModelSIM Simulator. Information available at `http://www.model.com/`.

[87] Modelsim XE Simulator. Information available at `http://support.xilinx.com/`.

[88] S. M. Müller and W. J. Paul. *Computer Architecture: Complexity and Correctness*. Springer-Verlag, 2000.

[89] Steven W. Smith. *The Scientist and Engineer's Guide to Digital Signal Processing, 2nd edition*. California Technical Publishing, Available at `http://www.DSPguide.com`, 1999.

[90] Xilinx Inc. *Distributed Arithmetic FIR Filter V5.0*, Core Generator, product specification edition, 2001.

[91] Answer record # 4427, Answers Database, Xilinx Inc. Available at `http://support.xilinx.com`.

[92] G. Even, S. M. Müller, and P.-M. Seidel. A Dual Precision IEEE Floating-Point Multiplier. *Integration, The VLSI Journal*, 29(2):167–180, 2000.

[93] Xilinx Core Generator, Xilinx Inc. Information available at `http://support.xilinx.com`.

[94] Micron SDRAM devices datasheets. Available at `http://www.micron.com`.

[95] Xilinx Inc. *Pipelined Divider v2.0*, Core Generator, product specification edition, 2000.

[96] Volume Graphics GmbH. Information available at `http://www.volumegraphics.de/`.

[97] Amdahl G. The validity of the single processor approach to achieving large scale computing capabilities. In *AFIPS conference proceedings, vol.30*, pages 483–485, Spring Joint Computing Conference, 1967.

[98] PCI bus interface for Xilinx FPGA. Information available at `http://www.xilinx.com/pci`.

[99] Xilinx Inc. *Using the Virtex Delay-Locked Loop, XAPP132 (v2.5)*, 2002.

[100] Xilinx Inc. *Synthesizable High Performance SDRAM Controller, XAPP134 (v3.1)*, 2000.

[101] IDT FIFO devices datasheets. Available at `http://www.idt.com`.

[102] N. Sorokin. Implementation of high-speed fixed-point dividers on FPGA. *Journal of Computer Science and Technology (JCS&T)*, 6(1):8–11, 2006.